What Must I Do to Get Well? and How Can I Keep So?

G. L. Simmons

Αριστον μὲν ὕδωρ

WHAT MUST I DO TO GET WELL?

AND

HOW CAN I KEEP SO?

BY

ONE WHO HAS DONE IT

AN EXPOSITION OF THE SALISBURY TREATMENT

Stuart, Elma

"If the prophet had bid thee do some great thing, wouldest thou
not have done it? How much rather then, when he saith to thee,
"Wash, and be clean?"

Fourth Edition, Thoroughly Revised and Greatly Enlarged

NEW YORK

WILLIAM A. KELLOGG

1889

B

TROW'S
PRINTING AND BOOKBINDING COMPANY,
NEW YORK.

TO HER

WHO WAS THE BEST AND HIGHEST INFLUENCE

OF MY YOUTH,

AND IS NOW THE MOST BLESSED MEMORY OF MY AGE.

WITH REVERENT DEVOTION, I LAY THIS LITTLE BOOK UPON

GEORGE ELIOT'S GRAVE.

PREFACE TO THE FOURTH EDITION.

I AM very glad that a fourth edition is called for so soon (the former edition of two thousand copies being sold out in less than two months), since this demand shows,—as does much private correspondence,—that my little book supplies a real popular need. It is essentially for *the People* that I write, the so-to-speak, uninitiated —not for scientists.

I feel very grateful to those reviewers who have given a kindly and friendly notice of my book; and yet, I could have wished that some had seen deeper into the philosophy and reasons of the treatment, in order to approach the subject,—so vital in its importance,—in a more serious, earnest, and larger spirit. The Salisbury Treatment—founded on the revelations of the microscope, and endorsed by the tests of chemistry—is no new thing, but has stood unshaken the daily trial of *years*. It cannot, therefore, be talked or laughed down. Truth—and this is truth—must at last overcome opposition. Harvey, when he promulgated his discovery of the circulation of the blood, had, doubtless, a good deal to contend with, in the prejudices of the orthodox medical practitioners of his day, who perhaps would have considered the answer of the Indian medical student in his examination paper on that subject, near enough, " It runs down one leg and up the other." Similarly, practical farmers found it quite impossible to believe, till shown by *actual* experiment, that water in wet land could find its way into *drains*, which is now the leading feature in modern scientific agriculture.

Some of my critics good-naturedly charge me with enthusiasm ; but when one feels deeply, can one write half-heartedly ? The mind that seeks to move others, must it not be " red hot behind the pen "—especially when every word that flows from it, owes its being to experience ?

Some medical gentlemen, especially those hailing from Scotland, have testified an almost needless ferociousness against my (I hope) inoffensive little book; which might have extinguished me, had I not remembered the highly conservative tendency of " the Faculty " in Edinburgh, as evidenced by their Medical School, which held its doors relentlessly closed against the admission of women as medical students, long after others had more generously opened theirs. And also, that a distinguished physician of the above-named city, gave, in my presence, as the reason for his share in " the barrin' o' the door," that he had seven sons, and therefore could not afford to sanction this wholesale invasion of his profession. Perhaps these critics of mine are similarly provided with their quiver full of these problematical blessings, and so " cannot afford " that their patients should be instigated to think for themselves in the prevention and cure of their illnesses. But I do not anticipate that they, nor any doctor, need feel much apprehension on this head; for my experience tells me that there will always be many cases where doctors, now paying *one* visit, will then have to pay *three*, there being great numbers of irresponsible people quite incapable of thinking for, and guiding themselves, who

will require under the Salisbury system of self-
denial for health's sake, so much constant per-
suading, scolding, cheering on, warning and exhortation, that doctors will have their hands
pretty full (likewise their pockets), ere the race
of the helpless ones becomes extinct, and, further still, *all* cases of serious illness will absolutely *require very careful and incessant watching* by the skilled physician and microscopist,
were it even only for the purpose of detecting
where the patients' performances are discrepant
with his promises, and of averting the consequences. For a salient point in the Salisbury
treatment is the easy detection of deceptions or
unfaithfulness in diet. When the patient does
not progress, or has relapses—*it is his own fault*,
he has only himself to blame. Either he has
not conscientiously followed out all instructions,—or he has tried to *improve* upon the
diet by the addition of vagaries of his own or
his friends' devising. This is a matter of such
positive *certainty* each time, that not only can
it be safely "sworn to," but may be equally
confidently and advantageously *bet on.* I am
amazed, at the audacity and illiberality that

can " pooh-pooh " so scientific and exact a system of investigation, and still hold on to the old, unsatisfactory fashion of " guesswork,"—at the unfairness which can treat this arduous, tried labor of years as a childish tale, even while withholding from it the test of an honest trial. It seems to me that the time has come—and none too soon—for *patients themselves* to wake up, and, in the interests of humanity and their own, demand a thorough, searching and candid inquiry into this alleged scientific method of diagnosis, prevention, and cure. If it should be found to fail,—then let it speedily and utterly be consigned to the limbo of impostures; —if, after honest and reasonable trial, it is found to be successful, and to bear out its statements and promises, let it be frankly and generally accepted. But to condemn it unheard, untried, is a confession of weakness, and an evidence of lamentable prejudice, wholly unworthy of the noblest and grandest of professions, that of Healer. This edition of my little book, is now, I am happy to say, being translated into French and German, and will appear in these languages in November, 1889. The first edition, in Ger-

man, had a pleasing success.   Also, I am proud
to say that a publisher in New York is, on generous terms, publishing this book in that city.

E. STUART.

April 20, 1889.

PREFACE TO THE SECOND EDITION.

THE origin of and apology for this little book, are the very many letters I received from friends, and more particularly from strangers, inquiring minutely about the Salisbury Treatment.

The answers took long to write (often was I thus employed from 5 A.M. till 5 P.M.), and after all I could not in the compass of a letter, indicate everything that from their questions I judged would be of use to my correspondents, in their endeavor to regain health or keep it. So this little book came to be evolved out of the needs of others, and I can truly say that I have put my whole heart into the work. And the abundant testimony that I did, and do still continually receive, to the *very great benefits* that large numbers are deriving from following the treatment as I endeavored to explain it in these letters, and in my first edition, has made writing this second one—if that were possible to me—doubly a labor of hope and love. More especially as I saw far greater possibilities for helpfulness and good, widening before me, on receiving from Dr. Salisbury his masterly work, newly published in America, " The Relation of Alimentation and Disease."

I begged and obtained his generous permission to use and make copious extracts from it. Accordingly, with close and deep attention I studied his book; and then very carefully rewrote my own; enriching it largely throughout with the fruits of Dr. Salisbury's wisdom, research and long and varied experience.

Knowing as I did for so many years what it meant to " eat my bread with tears, and lie weeping on my bed through the long night hours " in grief and pain, these pages have been written in the ardent desire to help others *to help themselves,* and save them from the suffering that I suffered.

I lay no claim to novelty, less than none to originality ; I have but done my very best to explain helpfully and encouragingly to the sick,

the beneficent operation of the Salisbury Treatment, as I have felt it in myself and seen it in
others, to explain it so clearly and practically,
that every intelligent man and woman may, by
its help, get well and keep well. This is the
goal towards which I have striven from my first
page to my last. And with this view, I have in
addition drawn attention to a few of the signs
easily discernible, *when one first begins to get
out of health*, so that the remedy may be adopted at once; and the pain, unutterable weariness, nuisance, and expense of illness spared.
Every word also that I have said from myself
is the outcome of tried and hard *experience*
learnt in conflict with a nine years' most se -
ere illness, and very much of it has been re-
called to me now by those inquiries I spoke of
above.

That words and experience of mine should
stir you to rise up and conquer back for yourselves health, and freedom from pain and
misery, as I have done, by the simple, sure and
safe means here narrated, makes me most truly
happy, and I feel—thankfully feel—that all I
have suffered and what I have written, are not

resultless. Nor for myself have they been altogether so either,

> " ⸺ all these years
> Of lonely being. I have grown
> To tenderer pity for the tears
> Of others,—gazing through my own."

ELMA STUART.

June 21, 1888.

HOW TO GET WELL.

MODUS OPERANDI;
OR, HOW TO SET ABOUT THE SALISBURY TREATMENT.

" Each truth, learnt from science or experience, must have become part of the man's existence ; the theoretical truth must form such a part of his very being that it influences, almost unconsciously, every practical action. If a theory of life is worth studying, let the propounder bring evidence that it has moulded his own character, has been the mainspring of his actions."
—KARL PEARSON, M.A.

-"Hundreds of thousands are dying, for the simple reason that they do not know how to live to keep well, or how to live to get well. Aside from injuries, infections, and poisons, all our ills are caused simply by doing what we ought not to do, and leaving undone the things we ought to do. It is painful to think of the terrible slaughter caused by ignorance."—*From a letter of* DR. SALISBURY'S.

THE question that I am asked oftenest nowadays, is " *What is meant by The Salisbury Treatment ?* " This question I propose here to answer to the best of my ability ; feeling it will do much to encourage and reassure those who are ill, if I can partly tell them how carefully, patiently, and wisely this treatment has been thought out and tried in all ways; what painstaking research, reasoning, logic, insight, and earnest sincerity were brought to bear on its discovery. If I can make the sick see clearly the reason why it has attained such success as a cure in all kinds and stages of illness, during a long course of years—nearly thirty-five—they will surely, for their health's sake, not refuse to try it.

Dr. Salisbury of New York, a thorough microscopist and chemist from his early youth, entered upon the profession of medicine in 1850.[1]

He was at once strongly impressed by the almost utter ignorance existing in "the Profession," concerning the real Cause of Diseases, and consequently by the uncertainty and haphazardness inevitable in the mode of their attempted cure. The dire list of so-called incurable diseases haunted his thoughts day and

[1] It is from the clear, unerring disclosures of the microscope, and by aid of chemical analysis that this treatment has been discovered.

night. He felt *convinced* that they must be curable since they could arise in previously healthy organizations, that there must exist a tangible *cause* for them, that the cause must be discoverable, and he resolved that he would never rest content until he had discovered it. I have no room here to tell of his long and arduous investigations, extending over many years, of all the means he used, microscopically, chemically, scientifically, both as to the human body, and the foods it most constantly consumes. Anxious, painful, and laborious were these first years; till at length daylight began to break in upon his persevering researches, and he found at last the clue by which he was to thread his way to complete success. Acting upon this glimmering of light through the obscurity, he began to experiment first upon himself alone, in the matter of diet, with vegetable and other foods, in undue proportion or exclusively; carefully marking the results and symptoms, and examining microscopically the passages, which showed how much of such foods did not digest but *fermented*, filling the digestive organs with yeast, carbonic acid gas, alcohol

2

and vinegar, affording therefore no nourishment
to the body, but establishing diseased conditions. Then, and at various periods of his life,
he hired robust strong working-men, four and
six together to live with him for a time, paying
them well. Without taking the exercise needful for health (which would have postponed the
crisis), they all fed alike, exclusively on the
vegetable or other foods on which he desired to
experiment. In this way he soon produced in
himself and them the various illnesses which
we, taking longer about it from more favorable
conditions and circumstances (exercise, partial
meat diet, etc.), produce in ourselves by pro-
longed unhealthy alimentation.

Among the vegetable foods on which they
all fed (one food singly at a time) were bread,
beans, potatoes, asparagus, maize, oatmeal, rice ;
and the other foods (also partaken of singly)
comprised beef, mutton, chicken, turkey, lobster,
fish, etc., of which *Beef* triumphantly bore away
the palm as the aliment most easily digested
and the most sustaining, and also as the food on
which, exclusively, we can subsist the longest
not only without injury, but with positive

good. After that followed mutton; and turkey
came in third, the rest being, for the purposes of
an exclusive dietary, practically "nowhere."[1]
He watchfully noted down all symptoms and results, and before he separated from his hired
men, cured them by a course of diet exclusively
of broiled lean beef, washing out systematically
the while with hot water. Some slight medicines were brought in as well; but, as Dr. Salisbury says, " they are merely aids to the restoration of healthy states, after the cause, or the
unhealthy alimentation, is removed." But since
he could not, as he naïvely says, carry his experiments on to the death-point with himself
or his "boarders," he bought over a thousand
hogs, so that he might test on them various
methods of feeding. (I may remind you that
the stomach and digestive organs of the pig approach more nearly the same organs in man
than those of any other animal. The digestive
secretions are very similar and act in a like

[1] Dr. Ephraim Cutter states that repeated experiments have
proved "that adult man can exist and thrive indefinitely on
lean beef pulp and hot water alone." That this latter is in itself also a food is evinced by the fact that we can, at a pinch,
sustain life, solely on pure water from five to eight weeks.

manner upon the food.) In order to be quite
sure of all his facts, he tended, fed, and when
they died, dissected them himself; and by
1858 he perceived clearly and unmistakably
that *all diseases not caused by accidents, poisons or infections, emanate from unhealthy
alimentation.* And having at last reached the
cause, the remedy was not so far to seek.
The occurrences and details of his labors and
experiments in this deeply interesting field
are given in his great work lately published
in America, " The Relation of Alimentation
and Disease," a work of vital interest, which
should be thoughtfully studied by everybody who duly values, and would learn
how to keep his most precious possession,
namely, his health. Dr. Ephraim Cutter, writing on the above experiments and observa-
tions on diet — says, that they were " careful, difficult, long, painful and thorough, and, I
speak advisedly—without a parallel in history:
and their results have removed some of the *op-
probria medicorum* of the past." And thus, in
1858, his life-mission opened itself out fully before him, and earnestly and with a deep sense

of responsibility did he set about it—not so much to make a living for himself as to help others to live—to endeavor to prevent disease, and to cure it. Nobly has he fulfilled that mission, as hundreds can now gratefully testify, who but for him would to-day be taking their long sleep in "the land where no man dwelleth," or would be as I was, hourly, for, eight and a half most weary years, sleepless, helpless, barely able to move, and night and day unceasingly suffering great anguish. If you who read these lines had but seen me then—could but see me now, after a few short months of the diet and hot water![1] Honor to whom honor is due. Let us then pay our tribute of praise and gratefulness, ungrudgingly, to the genius, solicitude, and unwearying perseverance that so long and carefully thought out and discovered for us this simple, efficacious, and safe means of prevention and cure of disease—Dr. Salisbury's Treatment.

[1] Two months and a half after I began the strict treatment, I could bend, and put on my own shoes and stockings, and lace and unlace my boots, which I had been unable to do for nearly ten years. And then, gradually, each invalid appliance and device, and all cushions, etc., were discarded:—and oh the *heartfelt* joy with which I saw the last of these nuisances disappear!

I now proceed to unfold the means of cure, and I find that it is not superfluous to say that I address myself to

THE SICK.

F you desire to get well, you will take four pints of hot water a day, and restrict, for a time, your diet to minced beef only.

One good hour, or longer, before each of your three meals, always on an empty stomach, take one pint of hot water,[1] as hot as you can *comfortably* take it, as hot as in fact your tea and coffee—that is from 100° to 130° Fahr. as it suits you best. *Do not try to take it too hot.* And some two and a half or three hours after your last meal, say, a good half-hour before bedtime, take your fourth and last pint of hot water. " The best times for the regular meals are 8 A.M., 1 P.M., and 6 P.M.; and the best times for taking the hot water are about 6.30 A.M., 11.30 A.M., 4.30 P.M., and 9 P.M." (*Dr. Salisbury.*)[2]

[1] For children—half a pint.
[2] Those who take their matutinal pint in bed—a good plan

The water must NOT be swallowed quickly, but *sipped slowly*, so as not to cause weight and distention. If you fancy, after trying it, that you find it " very hard " to take the whole pint at first, then it is very easy and permissible to take a little less to begin with, but I *strongly and earnestly* advise you to come speedily to your full pint each time, if you really wish to gain the whole benefit of the treatment. You cannot, in adhering to your pint, take an overdose ; *do not be afraid of it.* I take occasionally two pints at a time, and feel myself all the better for it, though I also thought a pint at a time rather stiff to manage at first, and only my conviction of the logic of it carried me through. In a very short while, habit, the great good you will feel yourself deriving from it, and its own soothing properties, will make it quite easy and even pleasant to you to take the full quantity prescribed, especially if you bring a cheerful good-will, courage, and dogged determination to your own cure. The keynote to this whole line

for everyone—should lie down on their *left* side for a while afterward, as this position facilitates "*raising the wind.*" Dr. Salisbury recommends this procedure.

of treatment, is,—*the patient* does his own cure,
not the doctor. Upon the patient's resolution,
perseverance and intelligence, depend the success of the treatment. The doctor points the
way, helps, exhorts, restrains, cheers and advises,
—and *the patient does* it,—or doesn't.

" It was only after repeated experiments that
the most favorable temperature, amount, and
hours for taking the hot water were determined
accurately as above given." Should you fancy
that the hot water " will make you sick "—or,
from the foul state of your stomach, should it
at first really produce some nausea, add to it a
little aromatic spirits of ammonia, a pinch of
salt, a squeeze of lemon-juice, or a little sulphate
of magnesia—nothing else besides. If your
mouth is dry and tongue clammy, lips dry and
hard, add to your hot water a pinch of chloride
of calcium or nitrate of potash, which will soon
afford complete relief from the dry, parched
sensations. Your tongue and mouth being in
this state, is a sure sign of a sour stomach,
and shows your urgent need of a good *scour
out*.

It would be well to take note of the fact, and

remember, that no beverage whatever, *quenches thirst* in the way that hot water does,

Some of the English doctors—especially latterly—prescribe hot water with, or shortly after meals. But this is to render its *raison-d'être* of very little or rather no effect, and to retard or impede digestion by diluting and weakening the gastric juice. The object and uses of the hot water, taken as carefully directed, are roughly these :—(1) It washes out the stomach thoroughly,[1] cleansing away all the sour yeast, slime, and mess left there after food, leaving it clean and quiet for sleep, and free for the action of the gastric juice on the next meal. (It is therefore easy to understand, with a very little thought, *why,* along with its other benevolent work, it soon cures indigestion, heartburn, and flatulence, and makes you very hungry for your food.) (2) It stimulates the liver to activity, accelerating the downward flow of the bile

---

[1] My son writing to me from his ranch in America, says, " An old miner to whom I showed your book, said, *It's good horse-sense,* and it's only nat'ral we should want a good *ground-sluicing !* " Ground-sluicing is a term in mining which means sluicing the bed-rock or foundation with water, until it is left as clean and smooth as marble.

through the right ducts and channels; and
when you remember that a man in health produces from a pint and a half to two pints of
bile a day, you will appreciate the importance
of not allowing this fluid to go " fooling around "
everywhere, to become re-absorbed into the
blood-stream, but of guiding it in the way that
it should go. (3) It causes a flow of urine
sufficient to keep in solution the uric acid,
which, when the urine flows scantily, so often
deposits as red sand ; and it renders the water
quite clear and pale in color, as it ought to be,
and consequently greatly eases the filtering work
the kidneys have to perform. (4) It liquefies
and purifies the blood, thus not only largely *increasing circulation and vitality*, and imparting
an unwonted sensation of permanent warmth
and comfort to the body, hardening it against
colds and chills; but (5) it greatly lightens the
work *the heart* has to do, making it much easier
for it to " handle "[1] the pure liquid blood, than

[1] See '' Hot Water as a Remedy,'' 4th Edition, 10th Thousand, price 4*d*. London, Simpkin & Marshall ; Lancaster, E.
& J. Milner. A very valuable pamphlet, whose compiler has
done generous and noble work in the Hot Water Crusade, besides being the first to make known the Salisbury treatment in

when it is sluggish, sticky, and congested. (6) It washes out the uric acid in the joints, which deposit causes in some cases, such as gout, rheumatism, etc., so much distress and helplessness, and keeps the articulations lissom. (7) It quickly diminishes pain, soothes and strengthens the shattered nerves, gives calm, cheerfulness, and strength to the mind, through the good work it does to the body; and (8)—boon unspeakable—it induces, thanks to a clean untroubled stomach, *sound refreshing Sleep.* It fulfils other beneficent offices[1] for the suffering, as also for those in health who desire to keep so; for, well or ill, *everybody* needs an internal bath, more even than an external one, " even comparatively healthy persons find it of much benefit;" but what I have said is enough to show the reason why those who have seriously

England; to whom, for that, and ever ready kindness and helpful encouragement, I gladly own myself deeply indebted. In this little book are many authentic and most interesting cases of cure, notably one of *stone.*

[1] Hot water is very valuable as at once soothing and stimulating in fatigue and exhaustion; only, there must be two and a half clear hours *since,* or one full hour *before* eating; for food and the hot water should in no case *ever* be in the stomach at *one and the same time.*

tried it on the lines laid down above, are earnest
in preaching it to fellow-sufferers, and indeed to
all, and are ardently desirous that others should,
by its means, enjoy a like benefit with themselves.   For myself, from the inestimable and
unspeakable good it has done me, and the numbers whom I have persuaded to take it, I seem
now only to live to preach hot water, and also,
where required, the diet of minced or broiled
beef.

In all chronic disease, hot water is the foundation of treatment by Dr. Salisbury, and he, as
its discoverer, says, as the result of his long experience, that were he limited to but one remedy, that one would be hot water.   Let any
having doubts of its efficacy note the above, and
just try it.   The longer you take the hot water,
the more you will find the benefit, and you will
very soon begin to feel a great difference in your
condition.   It may cheer and help you to get
down the full four pints a day, to be told from
the solid experience of another—namely mine—
that each pint you take brings you nearer to the
blessed goal of health once more : each pint
tells, makes for health, and that, even if you did

not wish to get well, in taking *regularly and systematically* the good hot water, you cannot *prevent* yourself from getting better and better day by day. Each meal of minced beef only, and each pint of hot water that you take, are milestones that you have *passed* on the road, and shorten the journey back to Health again. In reference to No. 4, my own experience may be encouraging to invalids. For many years past I have constantly felt cold, even near a blazing fire, east wind and damp caused me cruel suffering, and in summer I sat out only on the hottest days, in the sun, shivering with cold, though wrapped in furs. As to an open window, the very sight of one terrified me and I fled;[1] and the gratuitous alacrity with which I took very serious chills would have been laudable in a better cause. This winter (1887-8), the first that I have been on the minced beef diet, they tell me has been a severe one. But I know nothing of it. I have often by day sat

---

[1] "I fled"—this is poetical. I *scuttered* off as fast as I could, hampered with a stick in each hand as props to a pair of very painful legs, as weak and limp as a sawdust doll's. *Nous avons changé tout cela!*

with an open window and no fire, have always slept thus whatever the weather, and walked and sat out of doors most days, by no means wrapped up, with deep snow on the ground. Dr. Salisbury *foretold* this happy revolution, last year in London, assuring me that if I *fed properly*, I should come to sleep on a snowdrift and be none the worse. I do not recognize in my present hardy self the poor, shivering, chilly wretch of but a few months ago. In illustration of No. 5, I may mention that I used to suffer a great deal from oppression and irregular beatings of the heart on climbing upstairs, when hurried or even slightly agitated. Not one trace of this remains. Almost immediately on beginning the hot water, these distressing sensations ceased, and have never returned.

Now for the second part of the Salisbury treatment, namely the regimen. It is a diet, while the necessity for it lasts, of entirely animal food—lean beef, chiefly minced. The *reasons* for this diet are very carefully and fully detailed later on, for it is so much more enheartening to the patient to be told *why* he must do such and such things, than to be left groping in the dark. The meat for this purpose should be from the round or flank, above the hock, which is richer, more juicy, and less expensive than the sirloin. The meat should be freshly killed, as it separates from the fibre more readily and can be more finely minced, or chopped, than when it has been hung or kept, as for steaks or roasts. The plan is to have the raw beef[1] finely minced by sending it through a machine three times. All fat, gristle, connecting tissue to be completely scraped away, (this can be utilized for soup if carefully skimmed); the mince to be made up very lightly and rather sloppily into cakes; seasoned with black pepper and salt sufficient to make them tasty; moistened with good soup, but not pressed hard and tight, as that renders them unpalatable and indigestible. The cakes must then be grilled well through, lightly on both

[1] It has always been a puzzle to me how the absurd idea originated, that Dr. Salisbury wants his patients to become Cannibals and eat the beef *raw!* Why, he even strongly objects to meat being underdone, as it is less soluble in the stomach than when *"done to a turn."* And, besides, it is dangerous to eat beef raw or nearly so, because of tape-worm, which is known to patronize beef, as well as pork and game :—an unwelcome tenant—not easily evicted.

sides, over a clear fire, turning the griller often.

N.B.—*No réchauffés allowed,* nor *cold* foods and drinks. If obliged to take them cold sometimes, warm them well in the mouth before swallowing.

The best griller (recommended by Dr. Salisbury) for these beef cakes as for the ordinary steaks and chops is the American griller. The American Meat Chopper also is far the best, as it cuts the meat, instead of tearing it.

Another way of doing the beef for a change, which is simpler, easier to cook, and which I like much better and find more easily digested than the beef cakes, is as follows. When finely minced raw (cleared from skin, gristle, etc.), seasoned with pepper and salt, and mixed thoroughly with a little good meat soup freed from fat and *used cold* (in the proportion of about a pint to one and a half pounds of *mince*), stir and press smooth with a wooden spoon over a gentle fire until *thoroughly, yet not over*-cooked. N.B.—*On no account must it ever boil,* as that makes it hard and lumpy, and thus detracts largely from its nourishing properties. (See

App. 3.) This is extremely good, easily taken, and digests and assimilates admirably; one does not weary of it, and you will soon be able to eat very plentifully, without any trouble, and to enjoy it. Several people have been kind enough to let me know that they also find this way of cooking the mince more palatable and easier of digestion than the beef cakes; and that they can take the mince thus prepared for months without its palling, whereas, against the broiled cakes " their stomachs rise " after a very little while. I imagine the reason of this is, that the beef cakes require much more careful cooking than they usually obtain, and I for one have long discarded them and have held contentedly and entirely to the mince, cooked simply in my own fashion, as described. Dr. Salisbury does not object to its being done in this way, provided no carrots, greens, grease, etc., are cooked with the soup used in mixing the mince.

If you find it too hard to manage the minced beef alone all at once,—the hot water, however, distinctly creates an appetite for animal food, and makes it easier to negotiate,—then, rather.

3

than give it up, take for a while, with each
meal, one or two pieces, not more, of bread cut
thin and roasted quite crisp in the oven. On
these you may spread a little fresh butter, but
you are not, on any account, to eat cooked butter in any form, or things fried in butter, grease,
or lard. Make the minced beef your principal
food, taking, say, four or six mouthfuls of mince
to one of roasted bread and butter. *Try, however, for your own sake to come as soon as you
can to the minced beef diet alone.* You may have
black pepper, salt, and mustard with your beef,
if desired, and a dash of chutney *sauce*, but no
vegetables except a little raw celery with each
meal, no made sauces, and no puddings, pies,
boiled paste, jam, vinegar (where you used vinegar, substitute lemon-juice—as in salads, mint
sauce, mustard, etc.), no pickles, cake, and so
on ; and milk, as an ordinary article of food, being very fermentative, is to be, as a general rule,
avoided.[1]

It is a hard diet, and fully exercises all one's

[1] "Milk contains a number of bodies which yield acidity by
fermentation." When taken by the sick at all, it should be
previously *boiled*.

force of will, self-denial, and perseverance; and
for that reason it is better to eat alone, or with
those on the same *régime*, so as to avoid temptation. For myself, I always find it considerably safer to *retreat* before temptation than to
resolve to get the better of it. That ends in its
getting the better of me to a dead certainty;
there is nothing for it, therefore, I find, but to
show " a clean pair of heels " when good things
are about—especially cake; and, therefore, I always eat alone. You see, the moral of eating
alone is just this,—that the first step in the
wrong road leads so naturally to the second,
and the second to the third, and the third on to
the thirteenth; so that the good gained in
weeks or months of hard self-denial and rigid
diet, is more or less undone in yielding to the
momentary temptation. In some severe illnesses (notably in diabetes), and in some stages
of an illness, the diseased condition of the digestive organs, caused by long fermentation, is
such, that a teaspoonful of sugar, or one mouth-
ful of fermentable food is sufficient to act on
them as a handful of " Mother " does when put
into a barrel of vinegar—it sets the whole in a

ferment, and the remedy has very much to begin over again.

Hence the burthen of all Dr. Salisbury's letters to me : "*Do not let one morsel of fermentable food cross your lips :*—if you do, you will
suffer for it and delay your recovery." I proved
the exact truth of this utterance,—not only *once*
alas! for I too have "experimented" a good deal
in diet,—not always, I fear, in the interests of
Science! I soon, however, found out *how right*
Dr. Salisbury was in all his rules and prohibi-
tions, and, at last, surrendered to the relentless
must, and heartily wished that I had been so
wise as to do it from the first. I also nobly
hand on to you gratis, another admonition of
his, given me when I wrote to complain of flatulence: "Don't overeat, and you won't have
flatulence." Brief, but to the point, and eminently sound! This rigorous diet has to be
continued as long as the illness lasts, but *great*
will be your reward if you pluckily and faithfully persevere, nor will it long delay.

If, being ill, in trust and confidence you adopt
this diet and the hot water, you are extremely
wise and very happy : and your recovery will

probably be one gradual but triumphant progress from first to last.[1]   As mine has been ; I was
desperately ill when I began the strict Salisbury
Treatment, I wish I could describe how ill, and
with what complications, in which most severe
gout and rheumatism, contracted muscles and
rigid joints, acute neuralgia all over me, dyspepsia and insomnia, each in an aggravated form,
played its evil part :—but I have gone right
ahead ever since, gradually, but steadily on the
mend, with no disheartening relapses.   I see no
doctors, take no medicines or stimulants, only
stick to my hot water and the minced beef diet
(both of which I have grown to like very much),
and report myself from time to time by letter to
Dr. Salisbury.

As to the quantity of food to be taken at

[1] I do not want anyone to be guided by mere Faith.   I would
not thank the keenest enthusiast led only by blind *unreasoning*
belief.   The Salisbury Treatment is a matter of clearest demonstration, it is not an affair of theory or arbitrary opinion.   In
this book I place the evidence of the Treatment plainly before
you : here I explain the laws of its working, and ask you to
searchingly weigh and try them ; and with the logic and reasons of it at your finger-ends, to take your stand bravely, seriously, sincerely, and from—not faith—but *conviction*, practise
and preach the good doctrine everywhere.

each meal, the rule is, *eat heartily*, always leaving off feeling you could eat just a little more. The Salisbury treatment calls not only for perseverance and self-denial in no ordinary degree, but it further exercises one's observation, judgment, *and intelligence.* For you need to very carefully watch that you eat as much as, and yet *no more*, at each meal than you can well digest, a point *very difficult* at first to arrive at; but necessary, in order to avoid blunders which would retard your progress. I am bound to say that I know no species of exhaustion so utterly *flooring* as that induced by an overtaxed stomach. The whole body is affected by it, and, for the time-being, the mind too, is a sharer in the general collapse. No one can judge in this matter so safely as the patient's own stomach. It is a mistake to try to eat by weight, by which I mean, to eat *up to* any special weight. You will soon learn to judge of the right quantity at sight, which is the safer plan. The strict diet is beef broiled or minced for breakfast, dinner, and supper (with the hot water as indicated). If hungry between whiles, take a sip of good meat soup, or a few mouthfuls of the minced beef, unless this should interfere with your hot water hour, in which case, take only the hot water, as it is a food and stimulant as well.

On adopting the minced beef diet so easily and quickly digested, you will, it is well to warn you, at first miss a good deal the filled out, pleasantly (aye, and sometimes mightily *un*pleasantly) " crowded " sensation afforded by the vegetable foods; and, therefore, in the night are apt to grow hungry ; or perhaps, the feeling is one of *exhaustion* rather than absolute *hunger*.

Do not try to go to sleep in that case. Your endeavor after sleep on an empty stomach, would be sure to end in failure. You would begin to think, then to worry over troubles that in daylight were quite bearable, but which in the silence, darkness, and your own exhausted condition become exceedingly black and grim. Always, as a regular habit, therefore have a cup of good meat soup, or a cup of mince (both covered) beside you, and take, when wakeful, a few mouthfuls of either or both, and soon sleep and oblivion will kindly enfold you.

A word of advice is absolutely necessary here, for those about to embark upon the

minced beef diet, and I beg to call their attention to it. *You will not get on as you should do
if you don't eat enough.* This point is of such
vital importance to the success of the treatment, and I have seen harmful consequences
follow the *not* eating sufficient, that I urge it
upon you very strongly. I think that where
you restrict your diet to mince *alone,* you
should try to begin with 1½ lbs. of *mince* in the
twenty-four hours. And do not neglect the
caution already given concerning the *habit of
having food by you in the night,* and to take
some of it *at once* if you feel wakeful; otherwise by morning you will find yourself wearied
and exhausted, when you ought to wake up
refreshed and light hearted, and *would* do so,
did you not allow yourself to run down for
want of food. It is in these *little things,* which
yet are not *trifles* I assure you, that the *intelligence* of the patient is of great value, and helps
him to watch his own case to good purpose.

It seems odd to me what a new idea it is to
so many people, that, when they lie awake at
night *thinking,* or are restless or have the
"*fidgets,*" nine times in ten, it proceeds simply

from *inanition* and consequent exhaustion; and
a few mouthfuls of soup and a biscuit, or a sand-
wich—if they had any of these things handy—
would speedily restore tone to the nervous system, and allay the restlessness, and the yet
more distressing fidgets, so that they could very
soon get to sleep again, as the effect of this
renovation. Men and women in even strong
health will allow Insomnia to become a disastrous *habit* for want of understanding the true
cause and the very simple remedy. Don't, if
you eat with others, be discouraged and abashed
if they look surprised and say, " What! are you
going to eat all that!?" To be sure you are;
and let them take note that while they have
the whole provision department comfortably
stocked (no corners left) with soup, fish, meat,
bread, vegetables, pudding, cheese, and goodness knows what besides—with liquids added;
—you have to satisfy your capacity on meat
alone, which takes up little room, digests
quickly, and for which your hot water has made
you uncommonly hungry. The rule for you
therefore is, mince *à discrétion.* It is not so expensive a diet as it seems, for it is your whole

menu, there are no extras. Dr. Salisbury says,
"You need not be surprised if the patient
comes to eat from two to four pounds a day,
and his appetite must be gratified." I began
with from six to ten ounces a day, I now make
short work of two pounds. But then I add no
other kind of food whatever, and I am, as the
result, so absurdly well, daily able to do and to
enjoy more—and the unwonted sensation of
buoyant health again, is more than delightful,
(Written September, 1888.)

Another word of advice and warning, is, my
experience tells me, greatly needed here, and I
earnestly speak it. When once you have *delib-
erately decided* to adopt this line of treatment,
impressed by its simplicity, common sense and
reasonableness, you will be exceedingly wise
to banish *at once and entirely* every vacillation,
doubt, fear; to keep your mind full of perfect
peace and tranquil hope, convinced that in
pursuing this line of treatment with no undue
haste and not without good reasons; you are
doing the very best for yourself that you know;
—and remembering always that results are in
other hands than yours. Leave them there in

quiet trust, and indulge all good hope with cheerfulness, which, if you carry out the treatment (either in its entirety or only in a modified form, as the case my require), you are assuredly entitled to do.

It is of supreme importance to you now, that body and mind should wholly co-operate and *help* each other, instead of pulling different ways. —"For the mind *helps* the body, and at times raises it, and is the only bird that upholds its cage."[1] Be, then, like the compass true and undeviating; not like the facile weathercock blown hither and thither by "I *wonder* if"—"I rather wish I hadn't"—"What do *you* think?" (who have probably never "thought" about it). All these waverings are very unsettling and distracting, and will surely retard your recovery. Away with them, they are unworthy. *Be at rest, hope, and trust.*

There are several points which I shall be careful to mention now, being anxious to omit nothing that can reassure and encourage you as you begin and continue the strict Salisbury system.

[1] Victor Hugo.

I therefore caution you beforehand that on
commencing the treatment in its integrity you
may expect to grow thin, lighter in weight,
look somewhat pulled down, and lose—not
flesh—but fat, and soft deteriorated tissue. Do
not take alarm at this symptom, and, thinking
it is all up with you, abandon the treatment.
Your friends and " the Doctor " will be sure to
say, " I *told* you so," wax doleful in their prog-
nostications of what is going to happen to you,
and try hard to persuade you back to the old
ways of physic and feeding. This decrease in
weight is really a good sign, not a bad one in
spite of appearances; and it is for you now to
show that you are made of the right stuff, can
stick to what is for your good, and hold your
own pluckily in the face of much talk.[1] I have
gone through all this myself, I grew even

---

[1] Your part now is bravely and rigidly to stick to the Treatment, carefully avoiding all fatigue in all ways, reserve your
strength, it is little enough you have ; and soon you will begin,
gradually but very markedly, to feel all your old self again.
Don't you be *downed* by your own fears or by other peoples'.
You are on the right road, and you will arrive all right at the
goal when just the first pulling down is over. Keep up your
heart in Hope, and be cheery and faithful. Everything depends upon *You.*

thinner and looked yet more ghastly thàn long
illness had made me; but though at first feebler
and weaker in body, I knew I was all right, for
besides my unshakable reliance on the logic of
the Salisbury Treatment, I grew clearer and
stronger in mind than I had been for years. I
have seen others in a like predicament, we came
out of it in triumph, and so no less surely will
you, however direful the forebodings. And you
may tell your prophets of evil that Dr. Salisbury himself forewarns you of this change, in
these words. "Never mind the shrinkage in
weight, it is natural and *absolutely necessary*,
for the reason that those foods which upholster
or make fat, are the very ones which produce
the disease. The weight decrease is not at all
dangerous or alarming. . . . . The patient
will again begin to make new and firm healthy
tissue at a later stage of his cure, when normal
blood-making processes are fully restored. The
tissue with which he has parted—devitalized
and enervated—is no loss, and must give place
to that of the new order of things." Ere long
you will be conscious of a gradual but sensible
increase from heavier blood, muscle, nerve, and

bone. You will find that you will gain in flesh and weight up to the necessary point for health, and if you *feed properly*, thereabouts you will remain.

It is, however, very much to be deplored, when the patient's friends rashly endeavor to dissuade him from a mode of treatment, which such universal experience shows, and a little careful examination on their own part would establish scientifically, to be for his undoubted benefit.[1] It seems to me that it is a selfish, unkind, and unconsidered course of action, and that it would be wiser and worthier in them, to devote a little time and thought to the study of the reasons for the Salisbury system ; so that, if in the course of the treatment *his* heart fail or his feet weary, they may be able—true friend-like—to bear him up on the wings of reason and faith, and cheer him on to persevere in the good but sometimes difficult way. How sweet a little kindly encouragement is, in the midst of opposition and discouragement, none know better than

[1] I have seen people who scoffed at the Treatment, take very kindly to it themselves, in illness from which the usual remedies gave them no relief. I have seen many *converts*, I am glad to say.

I, nor how thankfully it is treasured in the comforted heart.

And again I give Dr. Salisbury's own note of warning. "In the first days of the treatment the patient ofteñ feels very feeble, owing to the absence of the artificial stimulus of fermenting foods ; *this also is natural and need evoke no anxieties.* A cleansing process is not *per se* a strengthening one, *but is needful* in order to prepare a basis for the requirements of real strength." You should not now take much muscular exercise, but should live a very *still life,* as quietly and placidly as you can, most carefully avoiding all fatigue. Dr. Salisbury at this stage (which is only temporary) advises careful and gentle massage and, if possible, *drives,* as providing passive exercise without exertion.[1] As soon as you grow strong again, of course take out-door exercise in moderation. Then would be the time for a tricycle, that sub-

[1] The right time for the delicate in health to take exercise, is from two to four hours after a meal. Earlier than two hours interferes with digestion, and may cause pain or uneasiness. If exercise be deferred till later than four hours, there is the risk of exhaustion from want of food ; this speedily diminishes the remaining strength, and then, it is all up with digestion.

lime institution for those of us who cannot afford to keep even a jackass, and who care to
take our exercise at first hand (or foot) not vi-
cariously.   Cycling, in bringing into play the
abdominal muscles, in quickening respiration
and the heart's action and increasing circulation, has a powerful effect, through pressure, on
the liver, squeezing out the flow of bile, preventing its dawdling about, and making it go
quicker, and in consequence of these things,
cycling is wonderfully exhilarating and inspirit-
ing and makes for cheerfulness.

Climbing steep hills has a similar excellent
awakening effect on the liver, and if you can't
manage a daily climb, take any chance that
offers to run up and down stairs rather than sit
still all the while; and divide twenty minutes
between a morning and night performance with
the dumb-bells.   It will be well-spent time for
man or woman, always guarding against over-
doing it.   From the first, as I hinted before, on
beginning the strict Salisbury Treatment, it is
almost wonderful how rapidly *mental* strength
returns, how very soon work becomes once
more pleasure and not toil, and what a keen

interest we take again in subjects and things from which we so lately turned with weariness and indifference, if not with positive aversion.

Again, there is another good symptom sometimes mistaken for a bad one, to the extent of frightening the patient into dropping the treatment, and I call attention to it in Dr. Salisbury's own words. " The passages from the bowels will become black and tarry, and rather small in quantity ·. . . this must be expected. These dark and sticky stools are caused by the washing down of the black bile, which has previously been saturating the system and been partially carried off through the urinary organs and sweat-glands. The black condition of the biliary secretions is the outcome of long continued fermentation[1] of foods in the stomach and bowels, keeping up constant reversed peristaltic action in the digestive organs, gallbladder, gall-ducts. . . . The smallness of

[1] "Ferments are a peculiar change which some substances undergo to produce vinegar, alcohol, or acid."—You can see therefore how injurious an excess of fermenting food may be to the interior economy, which is not intended by nature to be a yeast-pot.

4.

the passages is due to the meat foods being
nearly all utilized in nourishing the body."
The motions gradually lose their offensive
smell, though they continue black, sticky, and
"scrappy" for a long time, six or eight months;
all which proves how greatly this washing out
of the liver and bowels, and clearing the alimentary canal from fermentations were required.

Yet again, on commencing the Salisbury
Treatment, there is often just at first some
diarrhœa. This is caused by the now plentiful downflow of the bile into the bowels—its
proper place—and we should assist and encourage
nature to eliminate the objectionable materials
requiring ejection, by taking a mild laxative.
As Dr. Salisbury says, "The cleansing process
is in itself right and natural, these matters must
all be washed out of the system." But there
ought to be no violent "scourings," and should
this diarrhœa continue *too long*, take a little
boiled milk with a good dash of black pepper in
it, or some cinnamon or ginger tea, and lessen
the quantity of hot water so as not to dilute the
tea too much; do not be alarmed, but *eat well
of the mince, and eschew for the time being all*

*unnecessary expenditure of strength. Remember
that all foods, drinks, and medicines which
heighten the color of the urine, or lessen the appetite for meat, should be avoided.* Clothe always warmly and comfortably, by day and
night, in elastic woollen clothing,[1] which, without overheating the body, should be thick
enough to prevent your suffering from changes
of temperature and weather.

On the other hand, again, you may become
constipated ; and this is the reason for it. You
have been for many years feeding too exclusively
upon fermenting foods : and the carbonic-acid
gas liberated in the fermentations *has partially
paralysed the bowels,* which were only moved by
this bubbling, boiling, working yeast-pot, which
passes the materials down through the bowels
by the accumulating gases, which—except what
may be eructed up from the stomach—have no
other way of escape.

[1] Jaeger, and other later inventions notwithstanding, I hold
to the old-fashioned soft and light Shetland woollen undercloth-
ing as the best. Being open in its meshes, it is warmer in
winter and cooler in summer, and always healthy, as allowing
freely for ventilation and evaporation. If cotton is worn, it
should be the " *Cellular* " and never close in the grain.

Now we come to the point. The gas has paralysed the bowels, through being absorbed, *and they are only moving off mechanically by the pressure from above.* When the fermenting foods are *stopped*, and the patient is put on lean meat diet, but *little gas* is formed, and there is no longer *the force from above* to push the refuse matters along. The result is constipation. The meat does not *cause* it, but simply shows you how much the bowels have been paralysed by former errors in diet. If the meat is persevered in, and simple laxative tonics used to help nature for a while, the normal tone of the bowels *is restored,* and they will move as readily with beef, as with fruits. In fact, whenever any food *loosens* the bowels, you may know it is fermenting; and you should therefore *avoid* eating special foods to make them act. The bowels should be kept so well toned up and in such good working order, that they will move naturally, without mechanical or irritating aids. When people *persist* in taking fermenting foods and fruits to keep their bowels open, the large bowels finally become a yeast-pot too, and after a while so thicken, as to cause running diarrhœas or consumption of the bowels. This consumption of the bowels is the last stage in vegetable dyspepsia. The victims are still curable. The cure lies in *stopping* all fermenting foods which are the cause of the evil, going on the *strict Treatment*, and using cold water injections every morning to wash out the lower bowel and soothe it.

The constipation you may experience on commencing the Treatment, need not however *alarm* you, as there is extremely little *waste* in the food you are now taking. But a gentle laxative tonic will be necessary; and the gentlest, best (and nastiest!) is Cascara Sagrada, in fluid extract, *not* tincture. Next comes fluid extract of Rhubarb, and lastly, of Senna. Just sufficient of one of these may be taken on retiring, to give a satisfactory movement the following morning,— a teaspoonful, more or less. If the dose has not proved enough, an injection of a dessert-spoonful of glycerine in two tablespoonfuls of water may be used in the morning and retained fifteen or twenty minutes. In chronic constipation, the right quantity to move the bowels once a day should be determined by patient trial, and this must be kept up every night steadily without a single interruption; lessening the dose gradually as the bowels regain tone. In this way constipated states disappear slowly but certainly: the cure requires time and patience. Avoid extremes, for one extreme leads to another: take the happy medium. Never *physic*, but never allow constipation to gain on you. Use, as it were, just grease enough to keep the carriage-wheels from squeaking, and no more.

You can, for a change, if you like, in temporary constipation, chew a piece of Rhubarb root, a bit the size of a prize pea, two or three times a day. Dr. Salisbury calls this "lovely." I can't just honestly say I think it *very* nice, but it is decidedly good for the wholesomes.[1] When you ask at the chemist's for genuine Rhubarb root, see that you get it, and refuse to be fobbed off with manufactured stuff. The genuine root is not very yellow, is light in weight, porous, and rugged in shape.

It is right that, on commencing the strict

[1] Several correspondents have been so good as to let me know that when they take the water pretty hot they are troubled with constipation, and they are all right when they take it cooler. I am obliged by this hint and tell it here, so that each

treatment, you should be prepared for these contingencies, that you should know the *reason* of them all, so as to take things easy and not let yourself be upset or disheartened by them, as might be the case did they come upon you by surprise.

Narrowly watch your own case with vigilance and intelligence; not relying solely upon the assertions of others, in a matter that so closely affects your own interests. The urine should be examined daily with a view to color, density, and quantity; it must be perfectly inodorous, the color of a healthy infant's, which presupposes in most cases the absence of bile compounds, and consequently that your nervous system is not being upset and damaged by its own waste products returning to poison it. It should be without sand or sediment on cooling, it should stand uniformly at a density of 1.010 to 1.015,[1] and never be above 1.020; and should flow freely at the rate of from $3\frac{1}{2}$ to $4\frac{1}{2}$

person may study his own idiosyncrasies in this matter, and by trying and *observing*, arrive at what best suits himself.

[1] A wise move would be to procure a Urinometer with case and jar complete. It is fragile but easily managed, and is very useful. Pure water stands at 1.000, but as there is little

pints in twenty-four hours. The skin should be moist and soft, the bowels act comfortably once a day, the appetite for meat be good, with no hankerings after forbidden food. Then you may be *well assured* that all is going on favorably within you; "digestion and assimilation are so far improved that blood is made faster than it is used up, and repair of tissue is going on." Recovery has fairly begun, and if you are careful of yourself and kindly taken care of by others, so as to avoid all untoward accidents, you will win the day and go smoothly on from good to better, until health crowns their endeavors and your perseverance. It cannot— such a change and building up as this,—cannot be done impetuously. Nature works without haste but without pause, slowly but surely;

space on the indicator, this is represented by o.—10, 15, 20, etc., follow. The best urine to take as a test for the specific gravity, is that which doctors call "the water of the blood;" that is, the first you pass in the morning before drinking your hot water, and before taking food. Dr. Salisbury considers that this washing down and cleansing process requires at least a six months' course of hot water; but I know also that he considers it wise to continue the *morning and night pints* to your life's end, were it only to wash out the continually forming mucus from the stomach, etc., and keep the whole interior sweet and clean.

and the Salisbury Treatment is essentially one that closely follows the calm, unhurried course indicated by Nature herself. To quote Dr. Salisbury again, " When you have cleansed out the system and purified the blood, keep them so, and hope all things. There should be no hurry. Calm, passive following out of all instructions to the letter, will insure the life and health of the patient, if, with soul and body enlisted in the good cause, he treads this straight and narrow way." This is, indeed, a grand adaptation of the *Co-operative* System, and you will find it to be so, more and more, as body and soul associated, reap the reward.

And what is meant by " following out all instructions," is mainly this—*to take your hot water regularly, as directed, and to feed upon the food least liable to cause fermentation, the muscle-pulp of lean beef.* Take *nothing else* whatever, for the time-being; except an occasional change to broiled mutton.

And now, having so honestly laid before you the least alluring side of the Salisbury Treatment, it is but fair that I should be allowed to throw into the bargain, into the scale with

Health, this fact, which will surely be a compensatory reflection, and make up to you somewhat for all the persevering self-denial you are exercising. The Salisbury Treatment (the hot water and minced beef diet combined) is a great beautifier and rejuvenator of the complexion. After just the first pulling down, as pure rich blood is made, and repair of tissue advances, the skin will gradually become smooth and clear, wrinkles and lines will disappear, the eyes grow bright, your cheeks will take on the hue and contour of health, and you will look prettier and younger, and *feel* younger too, than you have done for many a year. All this, also, I can faithfully promise you from a very large experience. The *temper* moreover, very perceptibly sweetens under the benign influence of the Treatment. This consoling fact should be taken into account by friends who are inclined to discourage its adoption. It is so much easier "to be good" when one is free from gnawing pain and incessant malaise.

I have briefly given the rationale of the hot water; I shall now proceed to show the reasons for the second part of the Treatment — the minced beef diet. But, for the better understanding of it, I must preface my explanation by a few words on the cause of disease; for to expect to cure illness, while entirely ignorant of its cause, is to be indeed as one who leads a Forlorn Hope. Let us hear Dr. Salisbury himself on this important subject. "*Improper alimentation is the predisposing cause of disease.* Alimentation may be classified under two heads— healthy and unhealthy alimentation. Healthy alimentation is the feeding upon those kinds of food which any given organism is designed to live upon, as indicated by the structure and functions of its digestive apparatus. Unhealthy alimentation is the feeding upon food which the digestive organs cannot readily and perfectly digest. What would be healthy alimentation for purely herbivorous and purely carnivorous animals, would be *un*healthy alimentation for man, since he partakes structurally of both the herbivora and carnivora, and belongs to the omnivora. By structure, man is about two-thirds carnivorous and one-third herbivorous;" or put it in another way, he is expected to be

judiciously omnivorous.[1] "As a general rule, we
have twenty meat teeth and only twelve vegetable teeth, while four of these latter, the 'wisdom teeth,' are poor apologies as grinders. The
stomach in man is a purely carnivorous organ,
and is designed, both in structure and function,
for the digestion of lean meats. The small
bowels . . . are herbivorous mainly, and
are designed to digest vegetables, fats, and
fruits."[2] . . . *Healthy alimentation would con-
sist in a diet of about one part vegetables, fats,
and fruits, to about two parts of lean meat,* by
bulk, not by weight. When food only is eaten
that digests and assimilates well, there is no
fermentation or flatulence in the digestive organs. . . . Healthy alimentation, or feeding upon such foods as the system can well

---

[1] I wish that some people *read* so that what they take in at
one eye didn't go out so fast at the other, for then they would
not so often say and write to me, that Dr. Salisbury and myself,
denounce *in toto all other* foods, and condemn the wretched
patient to a diet *for life* of only minced beef! Does a doctor
who advises *temporary rest* for an injured leg, condemn *exercise* wholesale? The cases are exactly alike.

[2] Please see preceding note. The average proportions of
meats *usually* eaten, is about one-twelfth the bulk of bread,
vegetables, puddings, etc.

digest and assimilate, is always promotive of health. Unhealthy alimentation always acts as a cause of disease. . . . This species of feeding overtaxes those portions of the alimentary canal designed for digesting this particular character of aliment, and *overtaxes them so far that the digestive process soon becomes imperfect*, fermentation gradually supervenes . . . and palpable disease soon results."

I beg you to note the exceeding significance of all these words, as a guiding light in our own hands. They show most clearly *the enormous part that DIET plays in the health or sickness of each one of us;* and also to what a very great extent, and how easily serious illness, delicacy, and constant small upsets *are preventable* by practical attention to the plain rules of health, and it is *everybody's imperative duty — yours and mine* — to learn and to obey them. All illness that is not the result of infections, poisons, or accidents, takes its rise in the stomach,[1]

---

[1] Not only *illness;* imperfect digestion and malassimilation are often the unsuspected primary cause of many an ailment for which they scarcely get the credit they deserve: e.g. premature baldness, asthma, deafness, failure of sight, wens, warts, corns, bunions, etc.

and from thence invariably attacks the weakest part.

" *The disease proceeds along the line of least resistance.*" Nature's laws are unhasting, but remorseless and inexorable, and effect most surely follows cause. What and how you eat —your own actions therefore, determine unerringly, sooner or later, what you have of health or the reverse.

Now *the meaning* of the minced beef diet is significantly 'this. It gives *the very greatest nourishment* along with *the least possible strain and labor to the stomach. Being already finely broken up*, and containing no useless, fermentative, or flatulent constituents, no hard, gristly, indigestible lumps, it is digested and assimilated with great ease and rapidity. ' It builds up healthy tissue and muscle to replace the degen-

---

[1] *The reason* for removing so carefully all fat, connective tissue, gristle and skin, etc., from the lean meat, is, that *they* are as apt to ferment and generate carbonic acid gas, as are the farinaceous and vegetable foods : and also that there are many diseases which are *specially fed* by those fibrous tissues, which can be *cured* by a continuous course of diet, strictly of muscle pulp of lean beef : and *return* on the transgressor reverting to his old habits of feeding. (Cancers and tumors are among these.) Dr. Ephraim Cutter pithily epitomizes the sub-

erated tissue and diseased muscle, the outcome of long, unhealthy feeding, which this rigorous diet, in conjunction with the hot water, starves out, breaks down, and destroys. In the same way also and by the same process, the mince and hot water get rid quickly, and with absolute safety, of a very burdensome ailment—*superfluous fat*. This diet of lean meat also *affords rest* to those digestive organs (the alimentary canal, bowels, etc.), which have been long and greatly overfed and overtaxed, and gives time *for the repair* of the diseased, partially paralysed states therein induced by fermentation and the formation of yeast-plants in the intestines, as in a vinegar barrel.

To sum up—the aim and object of this course of diet is to *exclude* entirely from the patient all foods, drinks, and medicines that tend in any degree to get the system, or any part of it, out of order; and to persistently *starve out* those tissues that, from being over and unhealthily fed, require starving until no shadow of the disease

just this,—" The yeast fermentation of the food, from the vegetable kingdom and the connective fibrous animal tissues, is best avoided by removing them entirely from the field of operation ; as one renders a gun harmless by withdrawing the charge."

remains, and at the same time to healthfully
feed those tissues that require nourishment, until the beautiful state of perfect equilibrium is
again restored to the whole frame, which is always the issue and infallible sign of healthy alimentation. Feed ·healthily, and you will *look*
like it, and what is more, you will *feel* like it.

Talking of fat,—I once ventured to remon-
strate with a very handsome man on allowing
his beauty to be spoilt by obesity. He replied
with an air of intense conviction : " It is in my
family, an aunt of mine was quite fearfully
stout, and in fact she died of it eventually."
We can detect the weak point in this argument,
and yet calmly accept for ourselves, consumption, gout, rheumatism, and many other ills that
flesh is erroneously said to be *heir* to, on the
plea that they are " in the family." *Then get
them out !* Napoleon's *Junot* said that the *An-
cienne Noblesse* of France were merely descendants, he, with his title of yesterday, was an an-
cestor. Let *us* then, be no longer descendants
of gouty, consumptive, unhealthy families—but
the ancestors of long lines of hale and sturdy
men and women ; it is ours to be so if we will,

and is mainly to be achieved by healthy alimentation for ourselves and our children.[1]

Be careful to leave five hours between each meal, and never eat when hurried, worried, anxious, cross, or over-tired. Wait, rest, and grow calm; you will then digest your food comfortably and be the better for it. You should always make it *an invariable rule to rest tranquilly and thoroughly for at least half an hour before and after each meal :* to rest as the man said he did in church, who " just laid his legs up comfortable, and thought o' nothin'." *Rest,* nowadays, is almost a lost art. The manner in which women rest, like the way in which they

---

[1] Very true is the aphorism, "Call no man (or woman) happy till he is in his grave;" and yet, it were wiser still to add,— *and his children are in theirs.* Until it is shown to what he brought them into the world and with what predispositions; how he fed, how trained them, if he loved them well and wisely ; so that with virtuous minds and healthy bodies, they amid the fret and wear of the world, could fondly look back—

> " Oft from life's withered bower
>   In still communion with the past I turn ;
> And muse on thee—undying flower
>   In Memory's Urn."

Then indeed "happy" Father, happy Mother, even in the invisible silence and darkness of the Tomb!

eat when there is no man in the house to cater for, is merely a self-deception !

A man *rests*. He sensibly lies in an arm-chair with his legs on another, his head thrown back,—probably a pipe or similar delight in his mouth:—and thus, with mind and body in complete repose—he profoundly contemplates the ceiling. But a woman sits down with her work-basket, with her household accounts, with a book, anyway, with something *to do*, and announces darkly that she " is going to *rest* a while " !

In the same fashion if the male individual is to be absent from a meal, "anything will do," and so she pecks at one trifle and another, and wonders afterward why she has a headache, or indigestion, or "a sinking." Ten to one she will heap obloquy on the weather, and end by hasti-ly declaring " Oh, it's nothing, I'm all right."

Mrs. Malaprop pronounced the ways of Prov-idence to be unscrupulous (meaning inscrutable) —I affirm that the ways of women incline to both, in what appertains to their own comfort and health. The recent writer in the *Nineteenth Century*, who strongly advocated an occasional day in bed of rest and quiet, was a very sensible

and a very wise man. Try for only half a day
sometimes, for the sake of mind and body, even
if you are comparatively young and strong.

If you have taken too much at one meal,
don't miss the next, but make it a smaller one.
Masticate thoroughly, especially vegetables and
farinaceous foods, when you come to take them
again. These latter absolutely demand *a very
great amount* of mastication from every one,
more so than animal food, even where, as in the
case of meals and flours, they are already finely
subdivided. This mastication is to ensure their
thorough admixture with the saliva, which in
vegetable foods is the first and a highly important factor in the process of digestion. On animal food the saliva has no digestive effect, while
vegetable foods are not digested by the gastric
juice in the stomach as lean meats are.

It is unphilosophical and unsound advice—if
I may be permitted the digression here—when
"great authorities" advocate the use of farinaceous and vegetable foods as diet for the feeble and aged. For besides that these slops and
messes are uninviting and unpalatable to many,
they are mostly *very hard to digest*, and are not

nearly, bulk for bulk, so nourishing and so sustaining as lean beef finely minced and tastily
cooked ; they also require far more mastication
for insalivation from teeth that are absent—or,
like some of us, have seen better days.[1]

Will the feeble and aged please to accept a little kindly hint from me here, and, while wisely
sticking chiefly to their animal food, have their
meat, poultry, game, etc., always *finely minced*
for them every day before cooking. I promise
them that in eating a good deal more of this
nice mince than of other foods, they will derive
the maximum of nourishment and comfort, with
the minimum of effort to the enfeebled digestive organs ; and will thereby ensure for themselves a longer life, sweeter sleep, and a brighter
time all round in this pleasant world, for taking
Nature's hint in the decay of their teeth, that
the stomach also is less strong for its work, and
would be grateful for a little friendly extra-
neous assistance.

[1] If we swallow our food before masticating it properly, we
don't have a second chance given us, like the respectable cow,
to have it up and chew it over again—but must bear the unpleasant consequences of having "bolted." The human stomach is not a mill for grinding food, that duty properly belongs
to *the teeth.*

To return:—Drop, as a rule, all stimulants;
you do not really need them, they will do you
much greater harm than good. They should
never be taken but in *very special* cases, and
then only under the wisest, most cautious
guidance. As those, however, who *perceive* the
very grave responsibility they incur in advising their use are rarer than a white blackbird, it
is better and safer to leave stimulants alone.
Wholesome nourishing food will soon supply
all the *real* support you need, without the ex-
hausting reaction which follows the temporary
excitement and fictitious strength produced by
alcohol. A very *Will-o'-the-wisp* it is.

To drink *with* food *is a pernicious habit,*
tending to indigestion, the formation of adipose
tissue, and general flabbiness, and is quite unnecessary; but if liquid is taken, the quantity
should never exceed six ounces, a small cupful,
since it dilutes and weakens the gastric juice,
making digestion slow and difficult. You will
find that having quenched your thirst an hour
beforehand, you do not require any liquid at
meal-time; but if you must drink then, take
and sip while hot, a cup of hot water, or of

good meat soup, or—if your nerves can with
perfect safety stand them—*but be quite sure
they can*—a small cup of weak black coffee, or
weak clear tea, that is without milk and sugar.
Always avoid these last two items, as fermentative, flatulent, and difficult of digestion.

If, however, your nerves interfere with tea
and coffee—as in neuralgia, gout; rheumatism,
and all nervous illness may well be the case—it
is far wiser and safer to drop them altogether
for a time, till you are well and strong again in
fact, and to take instead Crust Coffee—made
thus in America.　Bake in the oven to a very
dark brown, some thin slices of good stale
bread.　Roll or pound them fine, and keep
in a well-corked, wide-mouthed bottle or tin.
While a breakfast-cupful of water is actually
boiling, put into the little saucepan a tablespoonful of baked crumbs (crust coffee); let it
stand a few minutes, then pour into your cup
through a strainer, and sip while hot.　This is
really "grateful and comforting," and far nicer
than the flat, often sour, and often smoked
mess called toast water, and is easily made
fresh each time.　With a little complaisant im-

agination you can make believe that it is *café noir*, and it is really very pleasant as a substitute for afternoon tea, and is warranted never to upset your nerves!

Be careful that you never, whether well or ill, allow yourself to swallow any hard lumps of meat, or gristly bits; *put them out*, they cannot digest and assimilate, and *are bound* to do you harm,[1] as shown in the note on page 62.

On commencing the Treatment, do not, for every little pain you may have, and which could quite naturally be explained, blame the hot water and stop it, as I have known some impatient people do;[2] do not, as I have known uncandid persons do, lay the unpleasant results of indiscretions in diet to the score of the hot water, dropping *it* instead of the indis-

[1] Remember the old Scotch lady, who, on accidentally taking a bit of very hot potato into her mouth, *speedily put it out;*—and looking round on the astonished guests, complacently observed, "Had I been a fule, I'd hae keepit that in my mouth!"—and do you imitate her good example in regard to gristle, etc.!

[2] This is as reasonable as to blame abstinence for any ailment one may be subject to, after having left off alcohol. In each case the wish is father to the plausible thought. There is present *the desire* to adhere to the stimulant, or to give up the hot water.

cretions, to your inestimable loss ; for without
the hot water you may be tolerably sure you
would have suffered a good deal more than you
did for your imprudence.   Do not, because the
Treatment does not cure you in a week, turn
from it with railing and bad language.   You
who have been patiently swallowing harmful
drugs for many years, may surely hold on patiently a little longer, while the diet and hot
water, hand in hand with Nature, are silently
but steadily accomplishing the purifying and repairing work within you.   A lady from America, who has had great experience in witness-
ing the success of the Salisbury System, wrote
to me lately these excellent words, which may
be useful here.   " Some people are so inconsistent about improvement and recovery.   They
do not take into consideration the probable
years they were in getting sick, and the dilap-
idated condition of their system when they commenced the Treatment.   And this diet must
be a slow process to recovery, because it begins
from the very foundation and *builds up*.   But
when the patient gets well again he is really
better than he was in the beginning, having

more healthy flesh and having acquired an appetite for substantial food." *Above all, do not lose heart ;* the way you may have to retrace is long, toilful, and weary, I know ; there is no royal road to health, it is a struggle at best; the crawl uphill again is not so fast as the run downhill was; but progress, if you persevere faithfully, will be sure and steady; and health —earth's best blessing—will be your great reward.

If you ask me how long the Treatment should continue, I reply that, in the absence of more definite guidance, the exigencies of your own state of health must decide that question. If, at the end, say of two, three, four, or more months, you find yourself quite free from pain, with digestion good, appetite hearty for the meat which you eat with enjoyment, if your flesh is firm and healthy, your sleep sound as a kitten's, if you are bright and cheery, feeling well, with the urine pale, clear and inodorous, standing for some weeks unvaryingly at 1.015, and all other matters going on smoothly and pointing healthward, then I know Dr. Salisbury would readily allow you to introduce other foods, carefully and gradually, into your diet.

Always on the clear understanding, however, that lean beef, broiled, roasted, or minced will continue to be the chief feature in your menu —your *pièce de résistance.* You could then bring in as adjuncts or side-dishes, mutton, lamb, winged game, especially the darker sorts, sweet-breads,[1] poultry, fish, a soft-boiled fresh egg, baked potato, well-boiled rice, bread stale,[2] or roasted crisp in the oven, and such like. But always continue, even when quite off the sick-list, to eat relatively *two* mouthfuls *of meat* to *one* of the other kinds of food, and, as a general rule, avoid boils, stews, *and fries. Watch your-self* extremely carefully when you arrive at making the change from the strict diet, and should there be a return of pain or of any un-favorable symptom, come right down at once to the muscle-pulp of beef again for a time; and

---

[1] Take care, however, that the sweetbreads are slowly and very thoroughly cooked. Ten years ago I ate an underdone sweetbread, and it is such a vivid and painful reminiscence, that I have never even looked at a sweetbread since!

[2] If you have an enemy, keep the new loaf for *him.* Never touch it yourself. Dynamite is a joke to it, and it transcends

afterward you can gradually and tentatively recommence the other foods in moderation. Some alert and intelligent observation on your part now will not be thrown away, believe me. You may sometimes have a small bit of cheese, stewed prunes, or other compote, and fresh fruit, *as a relish,* but not as a food; sweets must be used in great moderation, and fruit should be eaten only after the first two meals, never at night. Dr. Salisbury allows one good cigar or pipe, for a man where it agrees, after each meal; and I think he allows ladies who are used to it and like it, on the same conditions, when well, one mild cigarette.

I have one last word to add to the Sick, then I bid them farewell and *better* than well; God speed their cure!

It is a message of cheer and good hope, and is in Dr. Salisbury's own words, and I transcribe it with great pleasure.

"If we have the knowledge and disposition to reform and to remove these causes [of disease], and we go into the good work with our whole hearts, eating and drinking as we should, *repair — even to perfect health—becomes a certainty.*"

TO THE SEEDY.

AVING hitherto addressed myself to the Sick, I have now a little word to say to the "Seedy," after which I shall add a few words to those happy beings —none too many—who are able to write themselves down as "Well."

Dr. Salisbury, in his book to which I have been so deeply indebted through all this pamphlet, says, "The first and most important knowledge of which a physician should possess himself, is a thorough and detailed understanding of all the appearances, symptoms, and conditions of the body which constitute a perfect state of *health*. Without this he is unable to determine, locate, and measure the derangements which constitute disease. . . . He should be quick to recognize the first departure of the system from normal conditions, as indicated by slight but unmistakable changes in blood,[1] urine, stools, and secretions. . . .

[1] Dr. Salisbury always makes it a point on first seeing a patient, to examine the state of the blood microscopically. In

He should not content himself with the recognition of established disease in its earlier forms, but should detect it, so to say, in embryo." I venture to think that this utterance of Dr. Salisbury's applies in a modified form to each one of us, for what could be wiser than to endeavor to acquire some knowledge of the physiological appearances and signs which determine a perfectly healthy state, so that we may be able quickly, and even at its very source to detect the first symptoms inconsistent with that state? No illness comes on quite suddenly, there are always premonitory warnings, however slight. I proceed now to mention some of these, and beg to call your careful attention to

my first interview, he at once bid me put my arm on the table, and with a long silver pencil-case looking affair, he gave my wrist a good prod. (It didn't hurt.) He then squeezed out a large drop of blood, which he carried on a knife-blade to his microscope. He summoned me to look too, but I was none the wiser, not knowing the aspect of healthy blood; only, he said, that if I followed the treatment faithfully, and had the chance again to examine a drop in a month or two, I would not recognize it for the same, nor, in fact, would it *be* the same. Of which truth I am well persuaded, remembering how the suffering, and the swollen veins gradually subsided, until the latter reached the normal, and the former the vanishing-point.

them. For instance, when you find your water begin to be *high-colored*, scanty, having an unpleasant odor, depositing a sediment or sand on cooling, and in density keeping continuously over 1.015, then take to your hot water *at once* —and see to your diet.

Again, if the motions are constantly too frequent, liquid, frothy and yeasty, are offensive, expelled with wind and colic, are too pale or parti-colored, instead of being evenly of a darkish brown as in health; or if, on the other hand, they are continuously dry, hard, causing a feeling of weight and oppression, are difficult—perhaps painful—to pass, you are not in a perfectly sound state of health. See to your diet and take your hot water. If you become habitually wakeful and restless at nights, disturbed when asleep, dream evil dreams, if you arise in the morning heavy, unrefreshed, perturbed, and causelessly anxious and uneasy, with a " nasty taste " in your mouth, headachy, with weariness in your limbs, if you are unaccountably irritable in your temper, gloomy or depressed in spirits from no tangible cause ; if you become subject to chills, constantly have cold hands and feet, have little or no enjoyment in your meals, lose flesh suddenly, begin to be conscious of discomfort, distention, heartburn, or actual pain after food; many, or some only, of these sensations combined, *continuously experienced*, you may take as pretty conclusive proof that all is not well with you, *that your health is on the break and wants immediate and careful looking to.*

Then begin seriously to consider your ways. Do not knock under at once and say it is "God's will" that you should suffer, or, "that you must be ill some time," or call it "Fate," or "Kismet," which it assuredly is not, except that Destiny is *our own* doing (or undoing). For at that rate you would be content to sink down into mental and bodily invalidism without a brave struggle against it, calling it Resignation, an easy and self-indulgent vice in many cases, and thus allow yourself to become a horrible nuisance to yourself and all around you. Resignation is often but a high-faluting term for sheer indolence of mind and body. Its true name is self-indulgence; or, if you want a fine one for it, call it *laisser-aller*. Energetically set about searching for the *cause* which produced

the bad effect. Fight hard for health : it is
worth a hard fight. Go back in your mind
minutely over your recent diet, especially in
reference to the adequacy in amount of animal
food, and the proportion of fermentable foods,
drinks, sweets, etc., ponder over all you have
eaten and done, and amend your ways. Pull
up, as it is called, in time, and take a course of
hot water in earnest, correcting your diet the
while. Do not despise the symptoms, because
they are what you call "slight."[1] Be thankful
that they still are so, for they will be the more
quickly and easily cured ; and many a grave illness is turned aside by the recognition in good
time of those "slight" symptoms which mean
so much, being the outward and warning signs
of an inward deranged condition. They show
distinctly that the human machine is not being
kept in good running order. *"Digestion and
assimilation are very poor, and consequently blood*

---

[1] If I could but have read the meaning of these ever accumulating, slight but significant first signs, ten years ago,
ah ! what long anguish I should have been spared, what heavy
expense, and all the humiliations and inconveniences of abject
helplessness. I should have thought its weight in *gold* a cheap
price to pay for this little book of help, had I been offered it,
in those sad, hopeless days.

and tissue are not made fast enough to keep pace with decay and disintegration." Take warning then and preventive measures in time, so as to get back as fast as possible to that blessed 'state of absolute unconsciousness of our body which we call Health.[1] A little careful watching of the water you pass daily, especially in regard to color, will teach you much that is valuable in the regulation of your diet and the conservation of your general well-being, and is quite worth the slight trouble, since prevention is always easier and cheaper than cure.

When I say, " See to your diet," I mean this exactly, for there must be no vagueness here. That if you are, or are beginning to be *really ill*, you could not do better than, nor anyway half so well as to come straight on to the *strict* Sal-

[1] The thing is this ; that when you are not in perfect health, you are not, as it were, on level ground, you are always on the slip, at the edge of a declivity. You may get along all right apparently for many months, until one day suddenly there comes some worry or upset, or a bad chill, or eating some flagrantly indigestible food, or there is a mental or bodily strain, and—over you go. Then, it is not to say that you may run down,—but you are liable to toboggan down—to switchback-railway down,—to greased-lightning down :—and, once down, oh! it is easier sometimes to row up the Falls of Niagara, than do struggle back to lost health.

6

isbury Treatment at once, without delay, till
you have quite recovered. *Stop the cause,*
which is the fermenting foods, drinks, etc., far
too excessively and far too long indulged in.

If you are only beginning to be " seedy " and
out of sorts, greatly *reduce* the vegetable and
farinaceous part of your alimentation, taking,
say, *three or four* mouthfuls at each meal of
beef or mutton, broiled or roasted (and lamb,
game, fish, etc., on the same terms), *to one* of
bread, vegetables, or pudding, of course avoiding pastry and rich greasy dishes and sauces, as
well as fermentable drinks ; and always making
your last meal at night an almost exclusively
meat one, if not quite so, which would be wiser
still.

Pray do not, if you begin to feel ailing, fly to
drugs, tonics, "pick-me-ups," which *can* only
make you worse, aggravating the evil and enfeebling the whole system.[1]   Almost all medi-

[1] I do not mean to say that drugs are *never* useful, but that
it is far wiser and safer to trust alone to diet, hot water, and
Nature, when we have to do with doctors who order medicines
in the airy, affluent, and irresponsible fashion of which I, and
very many others who have written to me on the subject, have
been the victims.

cines are in themselves very indigestible and
cruelly exercise the unfortunate stomach already
unable to deal comfortably with even good
nourishing alimentation. As to tonics—my sad
experience of them is this : as is the spur to a
jaded horse, so is a tonic to a delicate constitution, or in a weakened state of the nerves and
health. It makes you *do all you can*, but is unable to put any *real strength* into you, while
"taking it out of you" to the utmost. The
safest time, I should say, to take alcohol (" pick-
me-ups "), drugs, tonics, and 'similar abomina-
tions, if you must have them, is when you are
quite well, robust, and strong, and *able to bear*
being upset and knocked over; but even then,
be careful. Dr. Salisbury says in this connection, " Medicines alone will not cure disease.
They are merely aids to the restoration of
healthy states, after the cause or the unhealthy
alimentation is removed." " Remember that
the medicines cure nothing, they simply aid in
keeping the machine in good running order,
while rigid and careful alimentation is effecting
the cure ; an alimentation freed as much as possible from all elements which tend to form con-

nective tissue and fat, or to paralyse the parts."
"The medicines to be used are simply such as
are necessary to aid digestion and assimilation,
and to keep the bowels open once a day."

How happy are the healthy! There are two
little words that for many years past have
seemed to me to hold in their meaning and as-
sociations all the music of the spheres. These
words are *Health* and *Work*. Ah, and if you
add *Youth* too, you indeed strike a chord that
vibrates into space, charming the ears and warm-
ing the heart of those who hear it. All earth's
fairest happiness crowns the possessor of these
priceless blessings, Health, Work, Youth! and he
is (or ought to be) as a King in his own right.

N you who are Well, I urge emphatically do all you can to keep so; take
your hot water daily, in the way already stated, and for the reasons minutely given.
If business hours will not allow of the full four
doses a day, you can always manage the morning and night pints, and these are the most val-

uable. Do not neglect this if you care to preserve your health to a good old age. When
you foresee the probability of getting home late,
after one of those days of hard work, worry,
scrimmage, and pressure, now so common, order
—especially if you are not so young as you have
been—for your dinner beforehand, at least for
the meat part of it, not *a joint* after your fish,
but a good big dish of Scotch minced collops,
dressed alluringly, as in the recipes given below,
any one of which is, in itself, a "dainty dish"
and fit for a king—when in health !

Scotch Minced Collops, No. 1.—Put one pound minced
beef (raw) in a stewpan with a little cold water, or better still, cold stock well skimmed, and one onion cut
small, black pepper and salt. Stir and press with a
wooden spoon till thoroughly smooth and hot. Then
add not quite as much water or stock as will cover the
meat and stew very gently for one hour. To thicken
the mince one tablespoonful of ketchup, one ditto Harvey's sauce, one ditto flour, mix with a little cold water,
and add to the mince a quarter of an hour before serving. Garnish with triangles of bread roasted crisp in
the oven. N.B.—In all cases where formerly toast was
employed, it is best to use thin sliced bread baked quite
crisp but not too hard in the oven, for pea-soup, sippits,

eating with butter, and so on. I have observed about
toast, that what I swallowed as good flexible leather, by
some unholy hocus-pocus of the digestive organs became transmuted inside me into sponge, with almost
limitless powers of expansion. This recipe for roasted
or *biscuit-bread,* which is my own proud invention, is
a great success and very popular ; many of my "patients" telling me they find it so wholesome and nice,
that they will not eat toast again.

Minced Collops, No. 2.—When wanted in a hurry.
Prepare a little browning of cut-up onion fried lightly
in butter in your saucepan ; add the raw minced beef
previously thoroughly mixed with a little stock, and
keep stirring with a wooden spoon. Add more stock or
gravy made from the skins, gristle and waste bits of the
beef, and cook, stirring constantly for twelve minutes.
Black pepper and salt to taste. Either of these recipes
is nice as a curry for a change, and the minced curry,
or collops, as it is not for a sick person, may be made
from cold meat, beef or mutton. *No.* 3. A very nice,
tasty dish and digestible, is made by adding nearly a
third of bread soaked in boiling milk or stock, mixed
smoothly with the mince, flavored with pepper, salt,
and whatever else you like, made into cakes about an
inch thick, brushed over with beaten-up white of egg,
and grilled very thoroughly over a clear bright fire.
No. 4. One more recipe—and *this one* makes a nice
change *for the sick* as well as for the healthy. Cut the

meat about an inch thick, and grill on both sides lightly, over a clear fire ; not to *cook*, but only to give a nice *taste of the fire.* Then cut in strips, pass it once or twice through the machine, and cook—if for an invalid —as on page 32.

Make your last meal at night chiefly of one of these, or of broiled or roast meat, excluding fermenting foods and drinks as far as possible, so that there may be no disturbing element to interfere with your night's rest and quiet sleep. This light but substantial supper will produce in you a post-prandial feeling of buoyancy and cheerfulness, instead of the depression and irri-tability that often result from a *solid* meat meal taken when the stomach is already largely shar-ing the exhaustion and strain of the body. At-tention to this little hint will, I assure you, greatly ease your burden, promote undisturbed sleep, tend to prolong life, save you from head-aches, indigestion and *malaise*, and make you feel happy, cheerful, and benevolent, by the comfort it will give you. All this will be reflected in the happy faces of those about you, especially of your womenkind, and guarantee to your family (including the baby, the dog, and the cat), a good time all round. The same dietetic suggestion applies to animal food eaten in haste before starting on a journey [1]—*mince it.* Many a sudden death is caused—as disclosed by the post-mortem — by hurrying, while the stomach is full of half-masticated, undigested, indigestible matter. Help it and yourself then, on these trying occasions, by sending down food already finely broken up. No man's soul and heart are quite in the right place, nor can he be reported safe and sound in health—whose stomach is overloaded and overworked.

"Man lives by what he *digests*—not by what he eats."

"Diseases enter at the mouth."—*Japanese Proverb.*

"The keys of life and death are in the stomach." —*The Rev. Ward Beecher.*

When you have passed the prime of life, it is much safer to let your train or 'bus go on without you, than to run the risk of hurrying to

[1] Cold roast meat *minced,* and seasoned with mustard and salt, and put between bread (buttered or not), makes excellent and wholesome sandwiches to take with you on your journey, and are eminently digestible and no trouble to eat.

catch it; for by running you increase the strain and labor of the heart at the same time that you depress its power by anxiety and apprehension.[1]

I may add that I have received several kind letters from hard-pressed, busy men in London and elsewhere, thanking me for the suggestion of the minced collops and saying "what a good friend" it proves to them two or three times a week when they get home late, "body and brain quite tired out." Nor do they neglect their morning and night pints of hot water, I am glad to say. You who are well, can do a great deal toward preserving your health, without the expense and risk of doctors, by carefully and intelligently watching the appearance of the water you pass. It should be, as we have seen, quite clear, and pale in color, "like a new-born infant's;"—and in quantity from two to two and a half quarts a day.

I hope you have remarked what has been said in this little book concerning the two-thirds

[1] Since this was written, I have noticed in one paper alone five or six sudden deaths from this very cause. Pause, before thus exciting yourself, and remember that *no return tickets* are issued on *this* line.

diet, as being calculated to *keep* well those who are so blest as already to possess their soul and body in health. A thoroughly healthy man or woman, one never having "anything the matter" with him or her, is in my experience somewhat phenomenal nowadays ; even quite young people complaining of insomnia, indigestion, neuralgia, and other ailments, of the very names of which I at their age, in the brave days of long ago, did not even know the meaning.

For your help in this important matter, health—I wind up what I had to say to you in Dr. Salisbury's words—"Nature gives us plain indications for our guidance in our natural structure—as fully stated elsewhere. We have twenty meat-teeth and only twelve vegetable-teeth, and the stomach (the first and largest organ of the digestive apparatus) digests nothing but lean meats, while the small bowels . . . digest vegetable foods and fats. We are thus about *two-thirds carnivorous* and *one-third herbivorous*, and if we live according to this structure—other conditions being favorable— *there need be but little danger of our ever getting out of order.*" Guard well then your best, your

most precious possession, since the keeping of
it is in your own hands.

The hot water alone, even without the diet
added, is the grand safeguard of those compelled to lead a sedentary life, through the want
of time and opportunity or the physical inability to take exercise. Let the sedentary make a
note of this, for should they be able only to
take even the morning and night pints regularly, they will very greatly benefit themselves
by so doing.

And in this place let me say that I do not
think it possible for a faithful hot water drinker
to become a voluntary suicide. The gloom and
wretchedness that give birth to that sad, un-
reasonable deed — "cet acte désespéré conçu
par la raison, mais exécuté par la folie" (the
only error precluding expiation)—are in a great
measure caused by the retention in the system
of effete matter absolutely requiring to be expelled; the product of undigested, unassimilable food, which the clogged system is not able
to deal with. Thoroughly flush the obstructed
economy with the hot water taken regularly,
throw and keep "the communications" freely

open daily and feed healthily. You will soon
again find life well worth living, and that your
own part in it is not so unsatisfactory and dis-
appointing as you perhaps imagined.

"Beware of desperate steps, the longest, darkest day—
   Live till to-morrow—will have passed away."

It would be well, too, if coroners' juries could
be induced to return a common-sense verdict
of unsound health, instead of the hackneyed
one of unsound mind, in most of these cases.
They would be speaking the truth, which in
itself is not a disadvantage, and at the same
time would read a necessary and valuable lesson
to us who remain, to look sharp after the small
first signs of a breakdown in health. When the
body is not in perfect health, it causes a condition of mental and moral uneasiness (often inducing cantankerousness) very hard to bear and
be borne with. And many wretched, impla-
cable quarrels, public and private, hopeless
misunderstandings between friends, terrifying
presentiments of disaster, melancholy and
gloomy fears, are due solely to indigestible food
pressing on some wrong place, or to a stopped-

up duct, which the diet and hot water would soon set to rights,—clearing the sluggish atmosphere, and—like Una—making sunshine in a shady place.

The hot water is also a certain cure for dipsomania. It eradicates the weary craving for drink, the overmastering passion for stimulant, and, in regulating the digestion and quenching thirst healthily and naturally, it drives out the disastrous hankering after liquor. This means has again and again been tried and found effectual. Even habitual drunkards have come at length to prefer the hot water to "drink."

And now I must be permitted to speak a little word to the hilarious and jocular, the facile jeerers, who, being of a certain calibre of intellect and a deplorable amount of prejudice, are much given to airing what they are pleased to consider their "wit" in the matter of the hot water and minced beef diet, on the scientific motive of which, and qualifications for prevention and cure, they are *profoundly ignorant*. Implying that it is a quack remedy, they style it a "universal" one, and declare it, sarcastically, to be "infallible." Well, I accept

the challenge, and I too declare Dr. Salisbury's
system, faithfully and accurately pursued, to
the utmost limits of such meanings, to be a
"universal" remedy and an "infallible" cure,
*in whatever stages and under whatsoever con-
ditions remedy and cure are still possible.* I
go further — I pronounce Dr. Salisbury's system, thoroughly and honestly carried out, to be
the grand *preventive* of disease; creating such
healthy conditions as render disease well-nigh
impossible, and that, I take it, is even better
than cure.

These are strong words, but not stronger than
the well-grounded faith that I hold, warrants—
not stronger than my now wide experience, and
the very plentiful *proofs* I have had, justify.
And if anyone will consent to use his common
sense and judgment and forego his "wit," looking calmly and judicially at the question, he
cannot fail to see that this whole line of treatment is a demonstration of the inexorable doctrine of Cause and Effect.

If there is some "good joke" here concealed,
I regret my destiny, while frankly admitting
my utter inability to appreciate—or even to see

—it. Do not, I beseech of you who are ill and in need of help, allow yourselves to be laughed out of what is of such intense importance to your whole life's well-being.[1]

When the strong are "out of sorts," and the sick are feeling more achy and feeble than usual, friends look kindly on, and sympathetically observe—often in good faith—"It is this wretched weather," or "It is this odious climate." Don't you allow yourself to be gulled by that. Except in peculiar cases, weather and climate have very little directly to do with it; but *errors in diet* have a great deal. Bravely and honestly face the fact, for please let me say that, generally speaking, we carry our own climate and weather within us, not without; and in feeding properly will become hardy and grow indifferent to both. And this is a merciful dispensation of Providence, or of Nature—since the remedy is thus not beyond our reach, but actually in our own hands. I do not say cli-

[1] The above does not in any way apply to good-humored banter, which is always pleasant and amusing, and he is a poor creature who cannot take *that* cheerily, especially as—"*Rira bien, qui rira le dernier !*"

mate and weather work you no harm once you *are* or *are getting* ill. But it is not in the power of the most malevolent east wind, or of damp, or cold; it is not in the power of grief, anxiety, or worry, nor of all of them leagued together, *to make* you ill. They cannot produce, let us say, gout or rheumatism. They can but induce conditions adverse to the expulsion of the uric acid, engendered by the unhealthy alimentation which is at the root of these illnesses. The camel's back, they tell us, is broken by the last straw. But "they" talk "bosh." It is what *lies under* the straw that causes the real breakdown of camel and health. The grief, the worry, the unfavorable weather and ungenial climate, they are the last straw under which, but for what has gone before, namely, unhealthy alimentation, you could have borne up bravely. No one has any right to die—bar accidents, before old age; and every one who does is either a suicide, involuntary mostly, or has been murdered by somebody's bungling. See all the sad and needless, early deaths in the obituaries; think over your own friends, young and in life's prime, alas!

" Whose part in all the pomp that fills
The circuit of the summer hills
——is that their grave is green."

A great deal of nonsense is also talked when invalids, especially great invalids, and with restricted means to boot, are induced to leave their comfortable homes and betake themselves to German and other Baths (where they are sometimes—as I was—terribly forlorn); often to their sore disheartenment, well-nigh despair, when they find they come back worse than they went.¹ The chief good, I take it, of these watering-places mainly consists in this: That

¹ Among the innumerable Baths and Health Resorts I was beguiled into trying, one stands out so dismally in memory that an account of it may amuse my readers.

The food was unwholesome, the baths cruelly draughty, the Medico a very rough diamond—all but the diamond—and the climate ungenial, damp and foggy.

One eccentricity of the place—and it really seemed to be upsetting—was, that of the sojourners there, hardly one could keep his or her clothes on for long together, let the weather be what it might. Were there a gleam of sunshine, off they all scampered to rid themselves of their hampering garments and luxuriate in a "sun-bath." Were it raw and dull, it was an "air-bath," with gymnastic accompaniment, again clothed like Cupid. And uncommonly "airy" they must have found it up on that housetop in the strong northeast wind that, even in autumn, frolicked so free over the plain. In all weathers, at all hours, on looking roofward, bare arms and legs were to be

7

people who are fairly well—well enough to have
been over-eating themselves and indulging
among other things in richly cooked, highly
spiced dishes, heated atmospheres, late hours,
and generally detrimental habits (in the back-
ground I am thinking, also, of those who have
added the strain of overwork to neglect of
other rules of health)—are put at once on a
plain, wholesome *régime,* undergo a good scour-
ing out by a course of daily internal baths,
drinking many tumblers of water with a fine-
sounding name ("What's in a name?"), either
hot or cold, but generally at a high natural
temperature.   They are made to rise and retire
early, to take plenty of active out-door exercise,

seen whirling in bewildering confusion, like the sails of lunatic
windmills.

   In my few short walks in the adjacent forest, I met the womenkind barelegged, barefooted and bareheaded, and the men re-
taining little but what decency exacts in this nineteenth century.

   Other of their ways were odd, and not very nice. At dinner
a Colonel in the German army rapturously devoured a dish of
large raw carrots daily. The sight was not appetizing, and I
thought this Teutonic Nebuchadnezzar should have been teth-
ered outside and his dish of carrots put down to him.

   I believe that if I live to be three hundred, I shall never forget my misery in that *Unspeakable Hole,* from the hurtful food,
chills caught in the baths, and, in a lesser degree, from its
rough queer ways.

many external baths, which open the pores of the skin and give egress to much impure matter consequent on a long spell of improper feeding. They almost live in the open air, and altogether experience a thorough *change* in mode of life, habits, diet, hours, skies, and language; and are thereby largely helped to repair the damage done to their constitutions. No wonder that they return home considerably lighter in heart, weight—and pocket, jubilant and elated, each one swearing by his own particular "cure." The great benefit to be derived from change of air, especially to a purer air—ways, food, people, skies, etc.—is by no means to be undervalued, but, in nine cases out of ten, people's best and cheapest baths—namely, internal ones—were singing cheerily away in the kettle on their own kitchen hob, had they but known it; and if they had sipped their hot water at home, used a little self-restraint in the matter of diet, and lived at all rationally, they could have taken their "change" for pleasure instead of for health, and might have wandered at their own sweet will all over the world, instead of being "ordered" to some special health resort.

To return to climate; to the sick, I would
say, as Dr. Salisbury said to me, "Live where
you feel happiest and most comfortable, only let
it be where you will have your hot water regularly, and can get really *good beef* for your
mince.[1] With this proviso, go or stay where
you yourself like best to be."

If, however, you have a home of your own,
I should strongly recommend your remaining
in it, at least until you are well again, for,
be assured that nowhere else can you carry out
the precise treatment so faithfully, comfortably and satisfactorily as in your own house.
I never could have attempted it — though I
longed to do so—horribly ill in a foreign hotel;
but that a lady, almost a stranger to me, pity-
ing my sufferings and grasping at once the
potentialities of the Treatment, most nobly
minced and prepared my beef diet for me, daily,
for eight months, at her own home. I wish I

---

[1] I did not realize the full wisdom of this advice until I lived
in Switzerland, and there daily demolished what was called
beef; but was just good honest *blanket :* tough, tasteless, and
woolly as a sheep's back.   It was skilfully cooked, I admit;
but, for the Salisbury patient—the Roast Beef of Old England,
and of America !

could raise a monument to her: but indeed *I
am her best monument*—a *walking* demonstration of her marvellous goodness, and of the efficacy of the Salisbury Treatment, I—who had
once paid a very grand doctor to come a short
distance to see me, six guineas, for the consoling intelligence that I " *must never hope to walk
again !* "

Dating from almost the *first day* that I was
able to begin the strict Treatment, the improvement in my condition *all round*, was so marked
and so steady, that *I did not dare to believe it,
for fear* there should be yet another terrible disappointment in store for me: and I felt that I
had had just about as many as I could well
bear.

Try hard to avoid all *fatigue*, whether from
any kind, inconsiderate visitors (a prolific source
of exhaustion and over-fatigue), exercise, work,
amusement, or any other cause, and everybody
should always work, exercise, and play *up to
their weakest point, not to their strongest.* As far
as is possible, take anxiety and worry quietly ;
to do otherwise can only knock you over, and
will cruelly undo in a few days the good you

have been slowly and toilfully gaining in many months.

You should put pressure on yourself in this thing, for the more you determine to take *the Inevitable*[1] easily, to be happy in your work and recreations, in your home and friends, and the more you feel a genial and comprehensive interest in everything going on in the world around you, the more perfect will be your digestion and assimilation, and the more healthy you will become in mind and body. Then, unless through accidents, there is no legitimate cause or impediment why you should not live, and enjoy your life for a hundred years and longer. If care killed a cat with all its nine lives, let us, who have but one, take right good heed that care shall neither extinguish nor shorten ours. Dr. Salisbury, lamenting our present waste of force and vitality, all too justly says, "We spend our lives in casting life away."

The hot water will help you well here, for it soothes the nerves and strengthens the mind;

---

[1] Even *argument* is lost upon the Inevitable. The only valid argument with an east wind is to hurry into your greatcoat.

so that cares and anxieties, which would have assumed exaggerated proportions and crushed you formerly, now sit far more lightly on your shoulders; you will find you have greater elasticity and courage to bear them, and can also *judge them more justly.*

And in this place, with all possible earnestness, I entreat and solemnly warn you, especially if you are ill or any way ailing, never to allow yourself to be ensnared by that calamitous blunder—that gigantic fallacy, *Vegetarianism.* Of all the gratuitous modes of flinging away precious health and inducing illness, this is about the foremost for rashness and folly. I speak from experience, for, regarding it as the ideal, humane, and perfect diet,[1] I anxiously desired to follow it always, and, to my life-long repentance, tried hard to do so six separate times, beginning more than eleven years ago. I carefully studied all its literature on which I could lay hands, I corresponded with and implicitly obeyed the guidance of some of its leaders, with this re-

[1] I still consider it all that,—only, unfortunately, there is wanting to us the *ideal stomach* necessary for its digestion and assimilation.

sult—that twice I brought myself so near death's
door that I heard the hinges creak, and still un-
daunted by that dire experience, tried it yet
four times more, causing myself very serious illness.   And but that I had, to begin with, an
iron constitution, nay, an adamantine one, this
wretched diet—unnourishing, because fermentative, flatulent, impossible of digestion and assimilation—would have had me long ago under,
instead of on the green earth.   I never yet knew
a vegetarian, and I have known many, possessed
of much real stamina.   He may keep well by
dint of hard labor, or brisk exercise and careful
living all round for a while, even for a long
while, I admit ; but when illness does overtake
him, *having no reserve of strength*, down he runs
like a clock with a broken mainspring, and his
resisting and rallying force, thanks to his inad-
equate nutrition, is lamentably weak.   It may
be " economical," as some count economy, penny-
wise and pound-foolish ; but the bill is high in
the end that we pay with doctor's fees and lost
health.   A "navvy " or a coal-porter may stow
away and be able to digest and work off the regulation amount of peas, beans, lentils, oatmeal,

etc., but for us more or less sedentary beings there are many far cheerfuller and more seducing ways of upsetting our stomachs, if we must do so, than Vegetarianism, and few—I speak feelingly—are more dangerous, chimerical, or so idiotic.

In considering diet, we must bear in mind that the nutritive value of a food must be counterbalanced by its digestibility. For instance, cheese as a force-giver possesses very high value, but its indigestibility reduces its nutritive worth to a very low rate indeed. The same remark holds good in regard to beans, lentils, etc. May I add that before eating green peas you should always mash them slightly on your plate to flatten them, for if you do not, many will slip down whole, in which state, of course, they cannot be digested.

When you eat salad, which should not be too often, cut it up small on your plate, and masticate it very thoroughly; and never swallow the skins, stones, or seeds of fruits, they are all insoluble, alien, *inert* bodies—not foods.

It may help to make the hot water a more welcome doctrine to you who are fairly well, to

know that you may now and then, with impu-
nity, "go for" something you like very much,
but which, unfortunately, does not like you. If
you continue to wash out well with the hot
water, an occasional treat will not much hurt
you; but be sure always to take the antidote.
Of the two great evils, eating too much and eating too little, the first is on the whole decidedly.
the least injurious, since Nature can throw off
superfluous matter, especially with the help of
the hot water, but she cannot create a supply of
the necessary food.

It is true of others besides *the poor*, that most
people do not eat enough,—enough that is, of
food the most perfectly fitted for assimilation
and to supply the wants of the body. Many
more die every year from under, than from over
nutrition.

The poor cannot get the right food, rightly
cooked,—the rich, while seeming to fare sumpt-
uously every day, yet consume mostly profitless
and incongruous futilities, that are not in any
real sense *food:* and starve in the midst of
plenty. We need not wonder therefore, that
an apparently trifling circumstance may cause

a complete break down, for we can bear so little on an ill-used stomach.

I give my own experience in regard to leaving off medicines, as I devoutly hope it may prove useful and encouraging to others.

Though very ill indeed at the time, I entirely left them off eight years ago (this was written in 1887), with exceeding benefit to myself. The way it came about was this : one of my doctors, intending to dissuade me from passing on to another, since under himself I only grew worse, told me that his mother had been a confirmed invalid and had died comparatively young, "solely because she had plenty of money to muddle on doctors," and he added expansively that a great authority¹ had said that "*Every dose of medicine was simply a blind experiment.*"² Like a flash my eyes were opened— the mystery was made plain.

¹ I read lately of another "great authority," who, on retiring from a large practice, gave as his reason, "I am tired of guess-

² This candid dictum of Sir Wm. Jenner's, reminds me of Voltaire's saying, that a physician is a man who pours medicines of which he knows little, into a body of which he knows less.

An appalling vision rose up before me of the whole chemist's shop I had, by doctor's orders, so confidingly and calamitously been swallowing in the last three years; and I no longer *wondered why* I had become so rapidly, desperately ill and dreadfully weak; when, at the commencement, I had suffered merely from rather bad indigestion, so easily curable by the hot water, had I but known of it then.

"Then," said I, "no one shall 'experiment' any further upon me, I have taken my last dose of medicine." I had rather a rough time of it with some, but I have held to my resolve—*to my infinite gain.*

In the early years of my illness, in my eagerness to get well again, I had over thirty-eight doctors of various nationalities, though chiefly English. After a long, long hiatus from the very hopelessness of finding any help among them all, by the greatest stroke of luck that ever befell me, I was told that Dr. Salisbury of New York City was in London. I will not speak of him, nor of the comfort, health, and happiness to which his treatment (the minced beef and hot water) has restored me, lest I be accused of

enthusiasm—a grave reproach in this age. The
other thirty-eight (among whom were five of
the brightest medical luminaries in England)
did for me, I imagine, their incompetent best,
some with willing kindness which I still remember gratefully; the rest (whom I don't remember gratefully!) in a very apathetic, half-hearted
way, discerning that the case was far beyond
them.' My slender purse became disquietingly
empty, but I suppose money, like the watch in
Bombastes, was "meant to go," and that is not
my complaint against them. It is this: that
they gave me, till I rebelled and would have no
more of it, day by day strong, cruel medicines
that still more reduced my feeble strength, de-
stroyed my health, my power to digest, and my
nerves, and enabled illness to obtain a mighty
grasp upon my thus weakened constitution.*

The case, though a very complicated and aggravated one,
was simple enough when the *cause* was exposed and checked,
as is fully proved by my progress from almost the *very first day*
that I began the Treatment:—progress, gradual, but steady
and perceptible.

I have kept some of the prescriptions still as curiosities
which, if they were not so sad, would be really too funny. In
most elaborate length are conglomerated together the most inimical, not to say warring elements, whose battle-field,
alas! was my luckless inside.

They should have *known* how much worse than useless was this mode of treatment, and if they did *not* know, they were ill-fitted for the high calling of Doctor. They bereft me of my health, and in so doing, took that which not enriched them, and left me poor indeed.

As to *diet* and its supreme and intimate relation to health and sickness, not one among them all had the faintest shadow of practical, available knowledge. "Keep up your diet," their stock phrase, meant, to my ignorant ears, exactly nothing ; and when I anxiously pressed for its precise meaning as a rule that I might obey, I found to my disappointment, that doctor and patient alike were floundering about in a quagmire of doubt and obscurity. But I forget ;—Two doctors had their ideas on diet, and here they are. One, the first I consulted of the thirty-eight, when I was in a low state of health from over-work and suffering from indigestion, was a very celebrated man indeed, and this was the daily *nourishment* he ordered me. Breakfast, 7.30, a rusk steeped in boiling water, water poured off and a little milk added. Dinner, 1, wing of a chicken or game, a little green vegeta-

ble, potato, bread, and a spoonful of a milk pudding. Tea, 6, same as breakfast. *Voila tout !*
and I " might safely continue " my long hours
of hard work the while.

In less than three weeks, this magnificently
substantial diet with the " remedies " added,
developed—to my bewildered consternation—a
terrible attack of rheumatic gout with great
weakness, which laid me prostrate for many
months with acute pain, helplessness, and total
disturbance of the whole system.

Another, honest man ! put his faith in eggs,
and set me on a raw-egg cure,[1] which was to
work me " wonders." I was desired to make
a hole in the top and suck the contents. This
I dutifully did, and I should be ashamed to tell
you the number I imbibed in a twelvemonth.
But at the end of over two years, having become quite *painfully* thin, exceedingly yellow,
and altogether very like a mummy, I realized
that, I had gained absolutely nothing but
greatly increased indigestion, and a dexterity in

[1] There is a hallucination existent that raw eggs are more
easily digested than cooked eggs ; but the fact is, that lightly
cooked eggs are much easier to digest than when raw, as well
as considerably pleasanter to the taste.

sucking eggs, that would have qualified me to instruct even my grandmother in the art. So I abandoned this wholesale slaughter of the (Alas! not always prospective) innocents, and sought elsewhere for the cure which evidently did not lie in an egg-shell.

Another doctor, by the way, saw my deliverance in brandy-rubbing. I was rubbed for an hour, daily, for many months, with good French brandy. This little entertainment cost me, in brandy alone,—exclusive of rubber and doctor's attendance,—just over £15. I only hope that I did "take it in at the pores," for it always seemed to me a quite sinful waste of good liquor. Besides, I felt injured that I should constantly smell so strongly of brandy (I was not allowed to wash it off), when I hadn't had one drop of it internally. This appeared to me hardly fair play!

Although I had had a good deal to do with bringing on the first stage of my illness by over-work and culpable unacquaintance with the laws of hygiene and proper alimentation (for of all that concerned health I was, eleven years ago, "as ignorant as the brutes that perish,"

without their judgment and discretion), I yet
showed one redeeming quality, had one wise instinct, and I tell it as earnest exhortation to all
whom it may concern, that it is safer to bear ills
of which you know the best and the worst, than
to add others to them the future consequences
of which you cannot foresee. My wise instinct
was this, and it undoubtedly bore its part in
finally simplifying my cure: I always firmly
declined to allow hypodermic injections of morphia, or to take any anodynes whatever to
soothe the excruciating pain that I unceasingly
suffered, along with almost entire sleeplessness
through many years. Doctor after doctor, in
pressing them upon me, protested that till I had
freedom from such great pain and some sleep, I
need not hope to be better; and finally they
waxed extremely wroth with me, and said I was
a most provoking and obstinate patient, which
indeed was true enough.

But my refusal arose from the instinct that
pain is a beneficent warning of danger, and that
in silencing that monitor you lull the body and
mind into a false ease and treacherous security.
Anything radically *curative* I would so gladly

8

have taken, but I despised and distrusted mere
palliatives, and I knew how morphia in all its
forms, and the other anodynes, upset one in
various ways, complicating illness; and that the
very paralysing the nerves and soothing the pain
which were to bring me comfort and sleep,
meant depressing my powers of resistance and
endurance, and enfeebling my mind. And I
knew besides, for I had seen it, the iron grip
which these counterfeit friends (opium, chloral,
etc.) are apt to take of those who have come
under their treacherous beneficence for relieving
pain and obtaining sleep.

I often thought I must go *mad* from the terrible longing for sleep and the still more terrible
want of it, from the anguish of pain from which
there was *no* repose, from the shattered nerves,
and the overwhelmment of helplessness and
misery. The very first night—years later—that
I began my hot water, I got three blessed hours'
sleep on end, and yet more sleep till morning. When I awoke I felt so happy I did not
know myself. And thus we have gone steadily
on, the Salisbury Treatment (minced beef and
hot water), Nature, and I, contesting the lost

ground inch by inch, until we have very nearly regained it all; and my condition to-day is healthier and sounder, my vitality stronger, and my sleep sweeter, than before I began sensibly to get ill at all, more than ten years ago. That is one reward for my "obstinacy," and the other I find in these words of George Eliot, "The highest calling and election is to *do with-out opium*, and live through all our pain with conscious clear-eyed endurance." So I say earnestly to my brothers and sisters in pain, Don't go in for "soothers," "pain-killers," lau-danum, morphia, chloral, chlorodyne, or any such poisons. You may have fierce pain to bear, but under the Salisbury Treatment pain is from the first sensibly lessening and becoming more bearable, as I can truly testify, until it goes away entirely; and in bearing it by the sheer force of your own pluck, at all events you are always assured lord and master of your own castle—your mind and body. Hold on bravely against all odds, and it will be the better for you, too, one day. N.B.—It is best to be explicit. The above does *not* apply in any way to anæsthetics or sedatives given for surgical operations, confinements, etc., or to bring tranquillity and relief at the last. These cases are totally different. My fight was for life and health, not for ease or euthanasia.

Apropos—Dr. Salisbury, by prescribing a system of healthful diet with the hot water, for some months before a confinement, reduces that interesting event, even when a first one, to a very slight and brief affair—a signal advantage to mother and child, and the whole household.

Miss E. J. Whately, writing to the *Spectator* of August 19th, 1888, mentions that a member of her family was suffering severely, when on a sea-voyage of some days' duration, from sea-sickness, and in hopes of finding relief took a cup of very hot water. "The result was immediately her falling into a quiet and refreshing sleep." Miss Whately here strikes a note in respect to the Salisbury System, that rings right truly. An American lady told me that for about a week before she started on her dreaded voyage to Europe, Dr. Salisbury limited her three meals daily almost entirely to broiled beefsteak, with the hot water at the usual times. A little bread baked crisp was allowed

with fresh butter, or some well-boiled rice, but
no sweets, puddings, pies, *fruit*, etc. Not being able easily to get the hot water on board,
she took a cup of weak clear tea with each meal
of roasted or boiled beef for the first two days,
and nothing else. After that she was able to
eat royally at the four generous banquets per
diem provided by the Company, and was, I believe, the only lady on board who stood to her
guns—I mean her victuals—with a healthy,
hearty appetite to the end of a very rough voyage. The rest, who had fed *gorgeously* at first,
dropped out of sight by twos and threes, and
their place at table knew them no more. I can
bear out this good testimony too, for never
since I have been a Salisbury patient have I
enacted the tragedy of Jonah's whale, which, in
the old days of promiscuous feeding, was with
me, on board a steamer with its various sounds
and sights of woe, an assured catastrophe. The
demon of sea-sickness passes us Salisbury patients by, and takes itself off to disport in less
healthy stomachs.

In treatment which deals so largely in Nature's generous gift to us of Water, it is of essen-

tial consequence that it should be pure and good.

If you are in a place where the water is in the least doubtful, or is hard, or is, as in Italy, Switzerland, and many parts of England (Dover, Margate, Dorking, etc.), full of chalk, then your only wise course is to send to the chemist for *distilled water*.   He has always more on hand than he knows what to do with, and ought not to charge you much.   (At Margate the chemist had the audacity to ask me threepence a pint for distilled water; at *Territet-Montreux* I got it from the chemist for five centimes a litre, i.e. a large quart for one halfpenny.)

Distilled water is always far and away the best water to drink in health or sickness.   It has very strong solvent properties, and acts powerfully on the earthy deposits and salts which are apt to accumulate in the system, and lodge there to our woe and the shortening of our lives.   It is also rapidly absorbed into the blood, and keeps the salts already there in solution, thus preventing their deposit, and also facilitating their excretion.

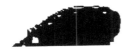

If you cannot procure distilled water, then I believe rain water is the next best, and by boiling it, its natural purity is much increased.

And now I shall endeavor to answer conclusively the objections often made to me in regard to the Salisbury Treatment. The first one very frequently made, is, " I must stop my hot water, for my doctor says it will injure the coats of my stomach."[1] " And does your doctor," I ask, " object on the same score to your taking your tea and coffee 'comfortably' hot ? " "Oh dear, no, not at all." In reference to this embargo of the doctor's, please give due weight to this fact, that the hot water *is a remedy*, and one that *is in the patient's own hands*. I know *great numbers* of people who have braved all these forebodings, and have found the hot water soothe and *strengthen* the " coats of their stomach " with the best results to their health. I can fully corroborate this testimony

---

[1] People have been so long used to paying their doctors to think *for* them, that when urged to think for themselves in the matter of care for their own health ; it seems an absurd idea which entertains *them*, but which they have a good deal of difficulty in entertaining, although it is high time that in sober earnest they should do so.

as regards my own " coats," which were in such
a feeble and irritable state before I began the
Salisbury Treatment, that for very dread of the
horrible pain I suffered for hours after eating, I
had brought myself down to one meal a day—
eaten in terror, and digested in torment. It is
greatly to be regretted when we, whose closest
interest it is faithfully and seriously to use what
of common sense and power of thought Providence may have conferred upon us, hide them
away in the napkin, and surrender our health—
and all that depends upon it—blindly to the
keeping of another.

And again, the sick say to me, " Why should
I go on the treatment, *my digestion* is all right ? "
But carefully read all that the treatment accom-
plishes in other ways, *besides* curing the pain of
indigestion ; and be sure, that, *if* your digestion
and assimilation *were* as perfect as you fondly imagine them to be, you would not be ill.
There are many forms of suffering and malaise,
besides local pain, in which faulty digestion and
nutrition reveal themselves ; for it is ever *at his
weakest point* that each individual is assailed.

The next objection often started is, " I can

quite understand how the Salisbury treatment can cure indigestion, heartburn, dyspepsia, and such like, but I can't understand how it should cure other and quite different illnesses, such as consumption, tumors, rheumatism, etc."

But there is no real difficulty *if you once for all grasp the fact, that illness, however varied its forms* (unless from poisons, infections, or accident), *is the consequence of unhealthy alimentation; and that the weakest part or organ in the individual constitution is the first to suffer.* Let us take a few examples and duly consider them, for the question is one of such great importance to us, that it fairly claims our most thoughtful attention. And while briefly advancing these instances, let me ask you to bear well in mind, that for over thirty years Dr. Salisbury has combated successfully, these various forms of (some of them) generally supposed incurable disease, in all their stages and degrees, by treating them as varieties produced by one cause, that cause being unhealthy and defective alimentation; and also, that by exclusively adopting that species of alimentation which the system is not able readily to digest and appropriate, he watch-

fully *produced* in himself and his " boarders," as
already mentioned, these very illnesses, and was
able *to cure* them when they were well pronounced, and had assumed grave proportions,
by systematically washing out the sour stomach
and bowels, and changing the food to such as
does not ferment and cause carbonic acid gas
with the resulting disorders. Dr. Salisbury,
with exceeding generosity, has given me largely
direct help in these following instances.

1. *Bright's Disease* is fatty disease of the kidneys. Now it is not possible to have fatty
disease of an organ until it becomes so paralysed that it cannot take up the blood that goes
to nourish it. In such cases Nature infiltrates
fat in order to preserve the tissue and prolong
life, long enough to give us time to remove the
cause and cure the disease. The cause of this
paralysis of an organ (the kidneys we are now
considering), is the constant and long-continued
over-indulgence in vegetable, starchy, saccharine
foods, drinks and fruits, which induce fermentation in the stomach and bowels, and keep them
constantly filled with carbonic acid gas. The
same foods also produce fat; hence in curing

the disease we have to *stop* all the foods and drinks that ferment, form carbonic acid gas, paralyse, and produce fat which feeds the disease.

2. *Diabetes* is a disease of the lobules of the liver. This portion of the liver is that which makes animal sugar. When we feed too exclusively upon foods that produce sugar (which include vegetable foods, fruits, animal fats, connective tissue, gristly bits, and so on), this portion of the liver becomes over-active, and forms more sugar than the system requires, and thus incites the kidneys to work excessively in order to carry off this sugar, and this over-strain of the liver and kidneys causes diabetes. By *stopping* all foods that make animal sugar, we lessen the activity of these organs, in time gradually bring them back to their normal state, and are thus able to cure the disease.

3. *Consumption*, which is a disease of the blood arising from continued unhealthy alimentation, is also to be cured only by removing the cause. This cause is fermenting food and the products of fermentation, sour yeast, carbonic acid gas, alcohol and vinegar. Any food that ferments with the acid yeast in the small bowels

may cause consumption of the lungs, and when in the large bowel, consumption of the bowels. To cure consumption we must stop the foods and drinks that ferment with the sour yeast, and these include all foods which ferment in a yeast-pot or vinegar-barrel; and feed up generously with the muscle pulp of lean beef, broiled or minced. The process is slow, as Nature's healing and repairing processes mostly are, but the cure is sure and certain, reaching even to those stages of this dreadful disease which have so long been deemed hopeless. The so-called *Microbe*, often advanced as the cause of consumption, is nothing but one phase in the development and metamorphosis of the various sour or acid yeasts. These vegetations, with the poisonous gases that are produced by their rapid development, cause both fibrous and tubercular consumption. And until the Microbe advocates learn and know what their "microbe" really is, *and how to produce and also how to starve it out*, they never will be able to cure consumption. (Dr. Salisbury's chapters on consumption in the work I have before alluded to, are of the highest value and importance.)

4. *Obesity* is a disease produced by over-feeding on the foods that make fat or adipose tissue. The cure is safe and simple. Stop those foods that make fat, and rigidly adhere, till the disease is cured, to lean meats, broiled or roasted, —beef, mutton, lamb, game, etc. (no great hardship!)

5. *Rheumatism* is caused by the too excessive feeding upon the foods that make acids. These acids, when absorbed to a certain extent, partially clot the blood, and make it ropy and stringy, so that when we expose ourselves to cold, the fibrous tissue round the joints contracts, which narrows the blood-vessels in those parts, and causes the ropy, stringy blood to hang in, and become dammed up around the joints, which condition causes rheumatic pains and excessive growth of joints. The cure is to stop all foods that produce acids by fermentation in the stomach and bowels, all starchy foods, and sugar therefore, and remove as much as possible the fibrous tissue and fats from the meat.

6. *Tumors.*—" All these fibrous growths and thickenings, and all excessive developments in

connective tissue where such development does
not normally belong, are the outcome of unhealthy alimentation." All tumors are developed in the fibrous, mucous, epithelial, and
bony tissues; generally they are in the fibrous
tissue. Any food that ferments in the stomach
or in the vicinity of an organ, forms carbonic
acid gas excessively, which is absorbed by that
organ so as to partially paralyse the blood-vessels of the part, and a standstill in the blood-
stream there is established; so that there is
over-nutrition of the parts under a state of partial death; and thus there is excessive growth
without pain. This process is one that makes
tumors. To cure these tumors we have to *stop*
all foods that ferment, and all foods that feed
the fibrous tissue. Dr. Salisbury says of these
diseases, as of cancerous growths, which are produced by the same cause, that " extirpating the
growth never removes the cause, and never results in a radical cure. The same wrong alimentation may develop still further and other
growths. . . . We must reach the underly-
ing cause before we can cure. We may relieve
and seemingly cure without knowing or re-

moving causes, but such relieving and curing is
not permanent. We should remember that all
these states and conditions *we bring upon ourselves, by something we are doing daily and persistently.* This wrong-doing must be *stopped;*
then we may use with advantage any means
that will help to gradually bring back and establish healthy states and habits in the diseased
structure." Words of highest import. If we
would only become thoroughly imbued with
the spirit that pervades them, what a shield
we should set up between ourselves and ill-
health !

· 7. *Neuralgia* is simply pain in partially dead-
ened nerves. This is partial paralysis, and most
usually is produced by unhealthy alimentation ;
although sometimes it may be either the result
of an injury, or some growth pressing upon a
nerve or nerves. Whatever the cause, that cause
should, if possible, first be removed, and then in
the second place we must restore the normal
life to the affected parts by *correct feeding* (the
meaning of which term you now well know),
aided by massage, passive movements, hot
baths, counter-irritants, etc., to bring the nour-

ishing blood and warmth back to the sick and weakened nerves. This disease, neuralgia, very readily yields to the correct treatment. Over-fatigue and general " run-down " make us an easy prey to this painful ailment. Add *Rest* to the means of cure (the diet and hot water).

8. *Dropsy* is not in itself a disease, it is only a symptom of disease in very vital organs ; and hence is not to be treated as a disease, but as a symptom merely. Dropsy in the extremities indicates disease of either the heart or kidneys, or both. Dropsy in the abdominal cavity indi-cates disease in the portal glands. The cause of the diseases that result in Dropsy, is un-healthy alimentation. The fermentation pro-cesses, with the resultant gases and other pro-ducts, are at the bottom of all these derange-ments. The same rigid diet and drinks are to be used in Dropsy as in Tumors and Bright's Disease.

9. *Pleurisy* is either inflammatory or neural-gic. Both forms of the disease occur in persons who are more or less out of order from indiges-tion. The inflammatory type occurs in persons who are able to make plenty of blood, but

whose digestive organs are filled to a greater or less extent with souring food. The acids developed in the stomach and bowels are taken up and enter the blood stream, where they little by little tend to make the blood ropy, stringy, and tough by partially clotting it. In this tough, stringy condition of the blood, any exposure to cold, or to other causes that contract the glue or fibrous tissues, lessens the calibre of the blood-vessels, and causes the blood to hang, or be impeded in its flow, resulting in a blockade and congestion of the parts affected, which is soon followed by inflammation. Now the great object in inflammatory diseases is to have *the most perfect digestion and assimilation possible.* The more perfect the digestion and assimilation, the more amenable to treatment are inflammatory diseases. In the neuralgic type of this disease—pleurisy—the gases developed from fermenting food in the stomach are absorbed with sufficient rapidity to partially paralyse the nerves about the heart, and often in other portions of the chest, producing partial death of the nerves in these parts. At a certain stage in this paralysis, the nerves begin to cry out in pain, to warn

9

us of the approaching danger if we persist in
eating fermenting foods.

In both these types of disease, fermenting
food, and the products developed by the fermentations, are at the root of the trouble. The
cure is to *stop* all fermenting food, wash out
well with the hot, or comfortably warm water,
and feed upon the nicest broiled or minced lean
beef or mutton in quantities that we can well
digest.

And finally, *Cancers are curable*, but they require such close attention, such careful watching,
that the patient would have to be under the
daily and most vigilant care of one who has had
experience in handling the disease. There are
so many little things to do in keeping the
moral, mental, psychic, and physical conditions
all in perfect balance, that the sufferer cannot go
on safely and successfully alone, as he very often
can, if he will, in other illnesses. The diet has
to be most rigid. The fibre has to be entirely
·eliminated from the lean meat, and this is a work
which requires very great patience and unswerv-
ing desire to have the food just right. The hot
water comes in as a necessity, and all parts of

the system must be kept in the most perfect order.

We have now gone carefully, though necessarily very concisely over many dissimilar kinds of illness, and naturally are much struck by the similarity of diet and treatment in cases apparently differing so widely from each other. But when once we entirely realize the fact that some form of *fermentation and decay* in vegetable foods, sweets, fruits, drinks, and the fibrous connective tissues of animal food, is either the producing cause of diseases, or the aggravating accessory (or both), it will cease to be a matter of wonder that, in handling them, the broad plans will of necessity be very similar.[1]

At the same time, however, a competent observer, closely following the symptoms of cure with open-minded intelligence, will soon discover for himself *where* the nice distinctive dif-

[1] I have been asked to add this short notice, which naturally does not belong here, on account of Dr. Salisbury's few words about the diet and treatment : " *Typhoid Fever* is produced by an infectious vegetation that develops in decaying animal matter in confined places, such as sewers, water-closets, etc. The treatment is by frequent baths inside and out, and a diet of lean meats, beef-tea and milk "—the latter should always have been *boiled.*

ferences occur in the mode of treatment, and the reasons for them.   Thus,—in the various fibrous diseases, Dr. Salisbury insists on the rigorous elimination of the connective glue tissues, skin, gristle, fat, and of all other fermenting foods from the patient's diet.   In diabetes, he forbids all foods that ferment and make sugar.   In Bright's disease, obesity, and all fatty infiltrations and deposits in organs and tissues,—all foods that make fat and are liable to fermentation, are strictly prohibited.   And in consumption, all foods are removed that are subject to acid yeast fermentation.

By closely studying the lines of treatment adopted in the various cases, the intelligent enquirer cannot fail speedily to become deeply impressed by the true scientific character, beauty and minute precision of the work, as well as by the simple logic and strong common sense of this essentially rational method of cure.

Another objection all too often urged is, "I don't *like* meat"—"I don't *like* hot water." This is simply childish, because when ill-health threatens or assails us, we may be certain that we have "liked," not wisely but too well, some-

thing or other that we had better have liked in
more moderation. Let me ask you, "Do you
like to be ill? Do you like your pain?" No?
then of "two evils" choose the one that is
not an evil, but a great good. I, too, in my day
"*liked*" bread and butter, jam, cake, cheese,
oatmeal porridge and milk, and puddings and
fruit much better than meat, and fed principally
upon them. But I have been taught in a hard,
stern school to like only those foods that like
me, and those are chiefly broiled and roasted
beef and mutton — animal food, in fact. But
the pleasant sensations of ease and comfort, the
glow and the feeling of health, lightness, and
bien-être generally (for want of an English word
to express it) that I now experience after food,
is far more than compensation for the old mixed
fare. Meat often gets the credit—quite unde-
servedly—of making us heavy, sleepy, and dull,
whereas it really is the "*bagging out*" of the
fermenting and flatus-foaming foods that gives
rise to those unpleasant sensations, certainly not
the meat.

And here I subjoin a significant *fact*, namely,
that I could, were I so minded, reproduce my ill-

ness with all its accompanying horrors of pain, sleeplessness, and helplessness, and not be long about it either, for I know the road well,— simply by returning to my former unscientific and unsustaining alimentation, discontinuing my hot water, and *eating between meals.*[1] And were I at the same time to resort to the genial assistance of Vegetarianism, and the kindly co-operation of medicines, then the rapidity of my relapse would only be rivalled by its stupendous folly.

Here is another objection very frequently made, and I grieve to say that it is not only quite young people who deliver themselves of this very foolish and unconsidered utterance, — "Oh, I can't be bothered attending to my health; wait till I'm ill; why should I trouble about it now?" I will venture to state the reasons why it were well to do so. First, because you are not the only person to be considered

[1] To eat between meals, even only half a biscuit, means just to set the whole machinery in motion that ought to be ab-solutely *at rest*, so as to be able to do its work thoroughly and comfortably at your next meal. Do not, therefore, disturb this necessary, beneficent repose; for, late or early, you will be the sufferer if you *continue* to do so.

in the matter; secondly, because attention *to health* is voluntary, easy, cheap, and painless; while attention *to illness* is compulsory, painful, difficult, and dear in all ways; and by disregarding the care of your health, you recklessly lay upon your home-circle anxiety, fatigue, trouble, worry, and expense, become a bore to your friends, and anything but a source of enjoyment to yourself—unpleasant results that are so easily avoided by a little good sense, thought, and unselfish consideration for others at the right time. " Sickness," truly says Emerson, " is a Cannibal that eats up all the life and strength it can lay hold of." It is absolutely selfish, heedless of what is good and great, afflicting the souls of others, and losing its own with meanness and mopings and ministration to its voracity for trifles. All successful men are Causationists; they believed that things went not by luck, but by law, and there is no *chance* in results. The first necessity is Health. " Get Health," says Emerson; and I make bold to add, When got, *do your level best to keep it.*

Some object to the hot water on the plea that " it doesn't agree with them somehow, they are not used to drinking much, are not thirsty persons:"—as if what they are *used* to do, or *thirst* had anything in the world to say to it ! The fact is, almost everybody is more or less subject to certain varieties of urinary deposits; and by causing much liquid to traverse the tissues, many otherwise insoluble substances are thus dissolved and washed away out of the system. If, however, *little* fluid be taken as a rule, especially if it contains solid matter (as thick soups, cocoa, tea and coffee with milk and sugar, etc.), this tends rather to increase the lodgement of deposits than to dissolve and eliminate them. If, therefore, those who offer the foolish objections above quoted, *had* been "used" persistently to employ this wholesome sluicing, they would probably have remained free from the various disorders, such as gout, rheumatism, calculus, and other uric acid deposits, to which people are subject who have "been used" to drink but little in proportion to their solid food. A wise doctor says, "even in health it is important to regulate the amount of liquid according to the solid matter of the diet." And, in reference to the maladies I have just named, he also has this significant word: "Notwithstanding all that has been said to the contrary, there is no doubt that in the cases we are considering, the most important part of the Treatment—and that for which no alternative or substitute can be found—is the administration of plenty of water." He would have been wiser still had he seen his way a little further.

I am often asked, "Why won't cold water do as well as hot?" Because cold water is apt to produce weight and discomfort, colic and pain. Nor does it act on the liver and bile as hot water does. It depresses vitality, and detracts from the heat of the body in its endeavor to raise the temperature of the water drunk to that of the blood, and this causes useless and even injurious expenditure of nerve-force. Cold-water bathing,[1] because of the drain on the nervous system, is also to be avoided; and likewise that insane practice of eating ices after a

---

[1] A soap and hot water bath should be taken twice a week, for cleanliness, after which rub energetically all over with a hard towel. Every night or morning sponge all over with warm water, in which put a tablespoonful of ammonia (liquid) to the quart of water. Rub well in, and dry vigorously with a hard rough towel.

full meal, chilling the stomach, which only digests comfortably to its owner at a temperature
of 100° Fahr.   Ice is valuable as medicine, not
as food.   Cold or lukewarm water, taken internally, never produces that feeling of *relief
and comfort* given by hot water, to which thousands of us can bear testimony.   In cases of
hemorrhage, however, the water should be
taken about 98°, that is, at blood heat.   In diarrhœa it sometimes does good to take it very hot
indeed.

Again, some people justify their rejection of
the Salisbury Treatment in illness, by saying
a little sententiously, " Ah, I daresay the treatment did *you* good, but *my* case is quite different."   First prove that your illness *in its origin*
did differ from mine, and then please take as
answer the last few pages on the various forms
of disease, all arising *primarily from unhealthy
alimentation;* and I think you will agree that,
in this instance at least, what is sauce for the
goose is sauce likewise for the gander.

Many people are afraid of the beef diet, as
being "too nitrogenous."   But first, beef does
not contain so much nitrogenous matter as

many vegetable substances do. This you can see for yourself in the following short analyses taken from Pavy, Fresenius, Knopp and others.

IN 100 PARTS.

Beans	30.8
White haricots	25.5
Dried peas	23.8
Lentils...............................	25.2
Dry Southern wheat [1]	22.75
Lean beef.............................	19.3
Lean Mutton	18.3

(While as to *digestion*, the first four require for that, at least an 80 wild-omnibus-horse-power.) And secondly; no one need fear to eat animal food freely, who unites to such feeding, its inseparable accompaniment, a thorough inundation with the hot water as directed. This completely averts any injurious effect; which fact, I, as a strongly rheumaticky and gouty subject, authenticate, who have lived and thriven royally, for very many months, on an absolutely

---

[1] By this you see that even your *bread*,—that part of it which isn't plaster of Paris and alum, may be more nitrogenous than beef. The statistics of the enormous yearly sale of alum in the rough to *Millers*, are truly alarming. *What do they want it for?* I have long known that many an unaccountable illness is due to *bread*, and I am not surprised at it.

exclusive, and for over two years on an *almost* exclusive meat dietary ; breaking its strictness only latterly, by, occasionally, as a great treat, taking with my mince for breakfast a small saucer of oatmeal porridge without milk, etc., and, more often at my dinner at 1.30, adding to the mince two of Mackenzie's wheaten biscuits and butter, with, sometimes, an apple, either baked or raw. (I should, however, be very sorry for myself if Dr. Salisbury came to hear of either the oatmeal porridge or the occasional raw apple—and, indeed, the latter I have been compelled to discontinue, for it I could not cheat, cajole, nor coerce my stomach into tolerating ; and as usual, on any difference arising between us, I had to go to the wall.)

That is all the variety I venture on, and I never weary of the regimen, nor does it weary of me. As one result of the beef diet and hot water, my complexion was never half so clear, smooth, fresh and healthy, even in my first youth—whenever that may have been.

Foster, in his large text-book on Physiology, says, that the most striking effect of a purely nitrogenous diet is to increase the metabolism

(change-creating) of the body. . . . "When,
therefore, a rapid renewal of the tissues is
sought for, an excess of proteid" (albuminous or
animal) "food may be desirable. It is possible
that an excess of proteid food, by reason of the
renewal of tissue caused by its metabolic activity, may be of service." (We know now that
it is something *more* than "possible.") And,
although in ordinary circumstances, an exclusive, or nearly so, meat dietary *would* tend to
overload the system with nitrogenous crystalline matters, yet you may, without the least
fear, and as conducing to *health*, adopt such a
diet, *while accompanying it* liberally with the
hot water, which keeps those crystalline substances in solution, hinders their deposit, and
ensures their expulsion in the urine. In this
connection, in "Foster's Physiology," it is written, "Water is of use to the body for mechanical purposes, not solely as food in the strict
sense of the word." And again, he says, "The
quantity of water which leaves the human body"
(which is made up of 75 per cent. of water) "by
the skin is very considerable. It is estimated
that while seven grains pass away through the

lungs per minute, as much as eleven grains escape through the skin. It has been calculated roughly that the total amount of perspiration from the whole body in twenty-four hours, might range from two to twenty kilos" (a kilo being 2 lbs.). Thus you cannot fail to perceive clearly the immense importance of hot water drinking to supply this perpetual deficit, and to preserve the tissues and skin, well-filled, plump, and soft, which otherwise become shrunken, withered, and dried up.

To drink the good hot water is, in another way also, to ward off old age; for it keeps the articulations limber and supple, and thus stays the advent of rigidity, that sad herald of senile decay.

It is often said to me in an airy, offhand way, "I don't agree with Dr. Salisbury about the beef diet; *I* think, or *my* theory is," etc. But it is no case of opinion, or question of theory; it is *fact*, and fact of long-standing proof; and you may just as well disagree with those who have proved that there is no such thing as color,—the fact is there audaciously, irrepressibly, just the same as if we had never differed from its propounders. It is a way facts have of making themselves unpleasant.

People sometimes say to me, "But I am obliged to give the patient 'slops,' for he will not eat solid food." *Then give him minced beef or "sloppy" as he and you like.* Reduce it to pulp in the machine, mix it very smooth and somewhat liquid with strong, well-skimmed, cold soup or beef-tea, cook carefully and slowly, stirring and pressing all the time, and make it tasty with a little pepper and salt. You may conscientiously assure the patient that in taking this nourishing, sustaining, health-promoting food freely, his illness will be shorter and less severe than it could possibly be on farinaceous and starchy "slops," and his convalescence will advance as if to music. It will not be the weary fluctuating process that convalescence is apt to be upon fermentable, flatulent foods. *Encourage him* by telling him this, for it is true.

Vary his mince often, making him tempting little dishes, and add sometimes for a treat a little mutton, lamb, turkey, game or chicken to the beef, and invent a change of amusing names for his menu—anything to get him to take kindly to his minced beef at first; for soon he will very gladly take to it, as he feels the ever-increasing strength and comfort it imparts.

In dealing with the sick it is good to remember how very limited his digestive faculty must needs be; and therefore it should be taxed only with what will *repay* the effort made, by affording the utmost nourishment to the patient. His power of digestion should in no case be wasted on futilities and kickshaws, but all economized for the right food that will be certain to give and maintain strength. "Avoid all foods that cannot be digested well, and give only those that digest *the best*." And long and careful testing has proved that the muscle-pulp of lean beef is that desirable food, being easily digested and quickly absorbed, and being never too heavy nor too rich for the weakest patient, as most people quite mistakenly suppose it would be. When liquid food only is expedient, beef-teas, carefully freed from fat, should mostly be given.

I lately saw in a little book by a doctor, a very sick man's diet-sheet which has since haunted me like a nightmare. The illustrious

Patient died on the 15th of June, 1888, and this was his day's nourishment on the 8th of that month.

"10 a.m." (It is not said if he fasted till then.) "Half a plateful of very thick porridge"—which is slimy, sticky, flatulent, and needs a great deal of mastication (for in-salivation) and of exercise to enable it to digest. "1 p. m."—only three hours after the porridge, which could hardly have been all disposed of—"Four eggs beaten up with wine"—Truly this was sorry nourishment and sup-port for a sick man, though four eggs are heavy enough, however well beaten. "Dinner"—(the hour is not stat-ed, but it must have been tolerably sharp upon the heels of the four eggs and wine at 1 p.m.) "Dinner, purée of chicken with mashed potatoes." A barmecide feast indeed for him whose utmost strength and resisting force were desperately wanted. Of all the vain imaginings that have deluded humanity, this of potatoes being more digestible because they are mashed, is one of the fool-ishest. A hundred times better, if you will give the sick an injurious article of diet, is a *baked* potato. You can be sure—a point for invalids of great importance—that it is thoroughly cooked, which you cannot be in the case of mashed potatoes, mashing being with many even good cooks considered equivalent to sufficient cooking. I have had repeated demonstration of this in severe indi-gestions therefrom. "In the afternoon a large piece of

10

cream ice and three eggs"—making seven eggs in one
day for a great invalid. Among the inscrutable dealings
of man with man, this "cream ice" is surely one of the
most bewildering and mysterious. The reason of it is
far to seek; the effect of it is not hard to understand.
"No supper," but "at 10 p.m."—when the patient
should have had his last *meal* at least three and a half
hours before, "at 10 p.m." he has "a large plateful of
shaped boiled rice"—a fermentable, flatulent, starchy,
compacted mass given to him whose stomach—worked so
continuously, although so erratically, all day—ought then
to have been clean, calm, and at perfect rest. *How could
sleep be his?* In the night, boiled rice, cocoa and eggs."
—More boiled rice, more eggs; and cocoa, which is always somewhat heavy, even when prepared entirely with
water. I could very soon *make* myself or another person ill upon such a diet.

Knowing from practical experience the supreme bearing of food on health *and on sickness,*
the above is almost the saddest, most pathetic,
record I have ever read. Tragic entirely :—
otherwise ludicrous.

And, great heavens! this is Science. I have
no hesitation in pronouncing it all, a futile, nay,
a starvation diet.

It is sometimes rather triumphantly said to

me that the Salisbury Treatment is " not scientific." On that point—particularly as no explanation is vouchsafed as to what precise meaning is attached to the word—I am too diffident to venture to pronounce an opinion. But I can confidently say for the Salisbury Treatment of illness, that if some narrow-groove men refuse to acknowledge it as scientific, it is notwithstanding thoroughly and undeniably *efficacious*, and the sick, I imagine, find that to be perfectly conclusive and satisfactory. May I, with submission, remind my critics that in the world's progress what is Science to-day may not be so to-morrow, as much of what was Science yesterday has faded in the brighter sunlight of to-day?

In short, Science, only a hundred years ago, would incredulously have scoffed at, as a lunatic's dream, half the common appliances of our present daily life—not to mention how aghast she would have stood at the high perfection to which we have now attained, in the scientific adulteration of everything, especially food and clothing. It is often said to me, " I am not ill, only seedy and ailing off and on [generally on]; will the hot water *alone* do me good ? " *Be assured that it will.* Can you thoughtfully read (pages 25-27) all the gracious services it renders, and doubt it ? Just try it. Give a fair trial to a good pint, even only morning and night regularly, if it is not possible for you to take it at other times too, and you will not be long in answering your own question very satisfactorily.

Again, I am frequently asked, " What is the object of *mincing* my beef when my teeth are still fairly good ? " But Dr. Salisbury does not unvaryingly prescribe *minced* beef for *everybody* in illness, only when the patients are greatly reduced in strength, and digestion and assimilation are much impaired ; *then* he orders a strict diet of the muscle-pulp of beef, as being very much easier of digestion and assimilation, rapidly absorbed, speedily utilized for building up the blood, and changing steadily all the body-tissues from a diseased condition to one of sound health. The mince, take note, also, is unworrying to the invalid in consequence of being very easy to swallow, when nicely and carefully prepared as it ought invariably to be. But when very tender steak nicely broiled, can be well masticated by a patient, and also well and easily digested, then Dr. Salisbury has no objection to its use in cases where fibrous diseases (such as tumors, locomotor ataxy, fibrous consumption, asthma and rheumatism) are not present, and where no enlargement of joints has taken place.

In all these *latter* instances *minced* beef or muscle-pulp, is always ordered, it being of the greatest importance to keep all connective tissue, fat, skin, and gristle rigidly away from the patient's food. To any one who has prepared the meat for mincing, or witnessed its careful preparation, it will be very obvious how the above-named substances are eliminated from the diet far more effectually than can be done by the patient himself in eating the solid beef, either broiled or roasted. And here I desire to bear my own strenuous testimony to the wisdom of adopting a diet of *minced*, in preference to *solid* meat, by the aged, or those not strong in health of any age, as *decidedly* tending to happier, easier, and longer life. An unspeakable boon, very simply obtained, and assuredly worth striving after.

Again, I am often asked, "What illnesses will hot water *alone* cure?" To which I reply that to take only *half* a well-attested remedy in a case of *illness*, is to trifle with your health and affront your understanding. Dr. Salisbury says, "*The hot water should be taken as prescribed in every case of disease, and forms an inseparable and valuable adjunct to this radical method of cure*" [the broiled or minced beef diet].

Again, he says, "Healthy alimentation, or feeding upon such foods as the system can well digest and assimilate, is always promotive of health : unhealthy alimentation always acts as a cause of disease. *Special feeding*, indicated by the condition of the system, acts as a means of cure in all diseases arising from unhealthy feeding." These few words will show you then, that it is not wise in the case of "illness" to divorce the diet from the hot water, since, so to speak, they play into each other's hands, and genially work together for your good.

Now, I am obliged to protest, that I never made for the Salisbury Treatment the preposterous claim that "it can work miracles;" but I do emphatically say this, and stand to it :—that to an outsider intelligently watching the cure when faithfully carried out, the progress made

by the sick on the strict treatment is very striking, and the readiness with which they mostly
at once respond to it, extremely gratifying and
encouraging. It begins *to tell* in various clearly
marked ways, almost from the first dose of hot
water, and the first meal of minced beef. Here
is no " miracle "; only, the result *one expects*
from this very rational and logical mode of helping our stern, but forgiving Mother Nature to
help us.

- The following are some among the diseases
which Dr. Salisbury *has proved* to arise, in the
beginning, from unhealthy alimentation, and
which *are cured* by his line of treatment. Consumption in all its phases, including chronic
diarrhœa, dyspepsia in all its forms, rheumatism
in all its varieties, neuralgia of all descriptions,
diabetes, locomotor ataxy, ovarian tumors, all
fibrous tumors, including uterine fibroids, and
cancerous growths. Many paralytic diseases,
softening of the brain, most cases of insanity,
many demented conditions, all forms of deafness, many diseases of the eye[1] and ear; all

[1] I heard an eminent oculist in London say that often he
was the first to tell many who were sent to him, after exam-

forms of gravel and stone, most kinds of asthma, all fatty diseases of the heart and other organs (except such as arise from injuries), anæmia in its various forms, most cases of prolapsus of the bowels and uterus, hypochondria, most cases of loss of voice, erysipelas, eczema, etc.

All these diseases, and many others, are simply the outcome of unhealthy alimentation, and by this, I repeat, is meant the too excessive and too long-continued feeding upon starchy and saccharine foods and drinks, and fruits, so that digestion *and nourishment* soon become imperfect; fermentation gradually supervenes, carbonic acid gas, which partially paralyses the organs, is produced, and disease eventually is, and must be, the result. The only real cure, is to *stop* all foods that ferment and paralyse and form carbonic acid gas in the stomach and bowels, *to feed* for a time *exclusively* upon lean meats, eliminating entirely from the meats all fibrous tissue, skin, and fat; and to thoroughly

ining their eyes, that they were but out of health, and that the failure of sight and pains in the eyes were only symptoms which would disappear when the stomach was restored to order. Doubtless many aurists could relate similar experiences.

and persistently *wash out* the sour stomach, bowels, and the whole system with the hot water. Dr. Salisbury further says that if we have the knowledge and the disposition to amend, and if we eat and drink healthily; repair, even to perfect health, becomes a *certainty.* Surely this promise, given after such long and wide experience, is encouraging and stimulating in the highest degree. I, too, can only say, to reassure and cheer on the fearful and doubting, that in every case where I have seen the Salisbury Treatment *honestly, and accurately* tried (in serious illness as in only slight ailments), I never saw the shadow of failure, nor have I ever heard of any failure, nor of anything but *out and out good* to the patient that came from adopting it; nor do I see, logically, how it *can* possibly fail. A valued though never seen friend, whose experience of the Salisbury Treatment is very great indeed, writes: " I have never known of any case where the treatment did any harm to the patient. Even in cases where the patient has no 'grit' to see the treatment through, he has always been benefited in his general health by his spurts of temporary adherence," and I also have witnessed the absolute truth of this myself.

People complain of the Salisbury Treatment that it is all very well for the rich, but useless for the poor who cannot afford it. I am very thoroughly ignorant of political economy, and my ideas on the subject, if I had any, would be quite out of place here. But I will just reply to the above objection that the Salisbury System points essentially to the *prevention* of illness, no less surely than to its cure;—and that if the poor would spend more on *Roast Beef* and *Mutton*, and less by several millions on fire-water and the poisonous adulterations which they call *beer* and *stout*, and would drink the good and cheap hot water instead, which increases the appetite for meat, and diminishes the desire for drink, there would be far less ill-health among them, far more happiness, leisure and ease; and fewer broken heads,—not to speak of the broken hearts.

I now come to a point which, though I have before alluded to it, I beg your leave to urge once more upon you *strongly*. Indeed, there are two points, and from experience and observation I hold them both to be of great importance. First, I advise any one suffering from *sleeplessness*, neuralgia, gout, rheumatism, indigestion, of all kinds, including sleep-walking, cramp, nightmare, sensations of falling, and so on, and from delicate health generally—even if such persons persist in rejecting the *strict* diet—while taking their hot water daily, as often as they can manage it; to make their *last meal at night, a meat meal entirely;* preferably of beef broiled, roasted, or minced, according to their illness, and their powers of mastication and digestion. And even those in comparatively fair health (especially those of us not growing younger), would be very wise to make lean meat, roast or broiled (which includes fish, poultry, and game), their *chief* food of an evening: because the digestive powers in nearly all cases, are weaker at night than at midday; and the lean meats digest very quickly and readily, and do not produce distention and flatulence, as other foods are apt to do. The evening meal while hearty, should be the lightest of the three. It is, further, very bad for " the wind," by which I mean the respiration, to go to bed either on a full stomach, or on one containing an undue

amount of fermentable food, such as bread, puddings, etc. A great deal of so-called asthma,
even in young people, owes its origin to this
latter pernicious practice. Let anyone try this
meat supper conscientiously *for a week or two
consecutively,* and he will experience a wonderful benefit. The gouty, and rheumaticky-gouty,
will find, as the result of a moderate entirely
meat meal at night (not forgetting their hot
water of course), that they are able, among
other good gained, helpfully and less and less
painfully to use their poor weak hands in the
morning, and similar advantages will accrue in
the other cases also, and even yet more abun-
dantly will the great gain be felt (almost at once
too) by the *Sleepless.* I am now morally certain
of this, that very many severe illnesses, in both
the young and the elderly, owe their origin solely
and entirely to a superfluity of fermentable food
and drinks at late dinner,—too much bread,
vegetables, sweets, fruit, etc., probably all together, *in undue proportion.* Then almost im-
perceptibly begin wakeful, restless nights.

From my own experience I can fully bear witness that the sleeplessness due to fermentation

is altogether a more distressful sensation, and
makes one far more wretched and uneasy, than
even that produced by too strong tea. The un-
conscious victim of fermentation soon has re-
course to drugs and sleeping draughts, which
cannot remove the cause, but instead, increase
the evil: for complications will ere long arise,
indigestion, constipated bowels, feebler health
and resisting power, etc.,—until it ends in a complete break down. I am speaking from my own
closely-observed experience, for I can now prog-
nosticate pretty accurately my night's rest from
my supper. With people that are in fairly good
health, it is not what they eat *occasionally* that
can hurt them. It is the continual dropping that
wears the stone away:—the continuously and
persistently eating the wrong food at the wrong
time, in the wrong proportion, that causes the
final disaster. I know not who invented the
stupid saying that bread is the staff of life, so
often hurled triumphantly at me in the sanguine
expectation of its discomfiting experience and
fact. Whoever it was, is as answerable in one
way for a good deal of the world's unhappiness,
as Solomon is in another, whose dictum respect-

ing the rod and the child, made of my child-
hood a misery at the time, and a pain to look
back on. But Solomon had more excuse for *his*
aphorism, since with his large family he must
often have been driven nearly distracted, and
constrained to lay about him with lavish pro-
fusion. Tea being the cup that cheers but not
inebriates, is another moonshine proverb.

We cannot, we who are not robust and very
strong, expect calm and undisturbed sleep with
the "risings" of a yeast-pot inside of us from
eating fermentable food at night. I repeat, for
the sake of the exceeding gravity of the possible consequences of continued sleeplessness, do
please, just give this a fair trial.[1] Many a fine
highly strung mind which runs off the rails
through insomnia, that all too common source
of suffering and disaster nowadays, *could be saved
by thus simplifying the supper or last meal.*

The second point is this : I hesitate to press
it, knowing the hardship of it, and that it will
be unwelcome advice ; I have not a doubt
though, that it is *good* advice from my own

[1] Bearing in mind the caution given (page 40) concerning
having food *get-at-able* at night, always.

oft recurring experience, and my observation of other cases. All those suffering from any of the above-named phases of illness, from weak nerves, nervous depression, any illness in fact in which nerves play even a subordinate part, will find themselves greatly helped to get better if they will *for a time, give up altogether tea and coffee*, and confine themselves, until stronger and sounder in nerve-force, to a little good meat soup, crust coffee, or a small cup of hot water with their meals. Tea and coffee have great medicinal value, and are, in æsthetic parlance, "distinctly precious;" taken on special occasions (by the delicate) they are splendid tonics, and don't do much harm: taken habitually, their effect is undoubtedly strongly deleterious in many ways, and notably as affecting *sleep, and nerves.*

I do indeed passionately desire for the health and happiness of my kind, that the Salisbury System and its proved truth, efficacy, and exceeding value as a logical, demonstrable remedy for illness simple and complex, shall soon be-

come a household word; for the accumulating
experience of every week, aye of every day, con-
firms me in the *profound conviction* that this
system of cure is the most efficacious and beneficent ever conferred upon suffering humanity.

And as practical recognition of its scientific
principles of operation and thorough straight-
forward success gains ground, illness in all its
forms, and with all its attendant wretchedness,
unless from poisons, infections, or accidents, will
gradually be expelled from the earth. This
is no Utopian dream, but a tangible Reality,
which is indubitable and indisputable.

I am told that I shall with unthinking people,
weaken the cause of the Salisbury Treatment by
what I have just said. But I do not write for
unthinking people, nor dare I conceal or modify
what I know to be a Great Truth, through fear
of what they may unthinkingly say. I write
for people whose lives are saddened and dark-
ened by pain and illness either in their own persons, or by seeing others suffer, and who, with
amazement, rack their brain day and night, as I
did mine, to find out *the reason of it all*, convinced that if I could get hold of that, I was on

the fair high-road to health again. Those who have kindly come with me thus far will, using their intelligence and power of thought, not misjudge the value of the Treatment, nor seek to controvert my statement, but will see that as we have stamped out the Plague or Black Death, and are endeavoring successfully to do the same by small-pox, cholera, and other epidemics, through everywhere creating such sanitary conditions as shall render these unhealthy states difficult, and finally impossible : so shall we individually, holding in our own hands the knowledge calculated to keep sickness at bay, eventually become exempt from those other illnesses which we now bring upon ourselves, and which mar and embitter and shorten our lives. As now we are the makers of sickness for ourselves, so shall we then be the architects of our own perfect health, and all lend a willing hand in building up that of our weaker comrades.

I am truly and warmly grateful to you, Friends and Strangers, who from reading my former editions, have so pluckily, and with fine faith and trust, gone in for the Treatment, to your "*great benefit*," as so many of you have

11

kindly let me know. I venture to think that you will find this more recent edition (thanks to the extensive "cribs" from Dr. Salisbury's book and the appendices, etc.) much more definite and useful in all its details, so that you can guide your own cases successfully to a cure by its help. The questions you have asked me, have also taught me a great deal in various ways; so true is it that the person who answers the question, is not seldom the one who is chiefly the gainer by the answer. Go bravely on in faith, in *certainty* of recovery. No man can hinder it if *you*, with your whole heart and soul associated in the good work, adhere to the right and avoid the wrong alimentation. In this, as in all else here below, you are your own best friend and helper, or worst enemy, and your dearest interest lies in your own hands. See to it that nobody, nor friend, nor doctor, succeed in dissuading you from the right path (alas for me this day had I listened to the dejected forebodings of either when I began the Salisbury Treatment). The pain and weakness are yours to bear, yours and not another's, if you return to the old ways of feeding that

wrought your affliction; if, for the future, you
feed in what has been shown you is the right
way, the good health, long life and welfare will
be yours no less; and the grave responsibility
of choice—rests with You.

HEALTH BE WITH YOU!

And now I close with once more a quotation
from the book which has so luminously eluci-
dated for us the Cause, Prevention, and Cure of
Disease. "From these experiments [in dieting
the hogs] we learn this important lesson: *Even
hogs 'cannot make hogs of themselves' with im-
punity, on a diet that the digestive organs were
never made to properly digest and assimilate.
. . . This fact is so vital, not alone to animals, but also in an even greater degree to
men, that I may be pardoned if I repeat, in
closing my work, Nearly all our diseases, aside
from those produced by parasites, poisons, and injuries in general, are the terrible outcome of defective and unhealthy feeding.* . . . It is my
abiding hope that *the People* may be brought
to see these facts for themselves, and may, by
individual and intelligent self-control, aid their

physicians to restore and maintain the oft-imperilled balance of Health. Without it, there is neither Beauty, Use, nor Happiness for us; in its absence all the great glories and truths fade away from our sick vision. . . . If we will not learn Nature's methods, she crushes us in the reversion of her laws, and passes on. But if we examine and inaugurate her processes, we become as calm and strong as she, and, like her, in our lives we receive and manifest the Divine."

Repetitions throughout this book, and unwonted emphases, have been really *forced* upon me from the novel aspect, strange and seemingly very hard of acceptation, that the Salisbury Treatment of Disease presents to many minds in England; completely upsetting preconceived notions, popular fallacies and old prejudices, which die uncommonly hard;—but, firm in confidence and trust, I joyfully look on to the time when all these shall have "melted away like streaks of morning-cloud, into the infinite azure of the Past."

No man can do better than his *best*, and I beg

to assure my readers that what I here offer them is, with all its deficiencies, my most anxious and painstaking best. For the subject-matter I in no way apologize. By every word of it I am prepared to stand, to die for its truth if need be, or,—what suits me better—while I live, to proclaim it.

It is my dearest and most ardent hope, to reach the minds and hearts *of the people,*—those who *feel* their sore need of help,—who, after many and bitter disappointments, are, as I was, *sick with hope deferred.*

May my little book then, spread far and wide, the knowledge of the powerful and beneficent Salisbury Treatment.

POSTSCRIPTUM.

I am driven to reiterate very clearly and distinctly, that from cover to cover of this book, I am advising, and speaking chiefly to the *Sick ;* and afterward to the off and on *Seedy,*—and that the few words I address to the comparatively *Well,* are for such as yet require to use *some* care, having to lead, through circumstances a more or less sedentary life,—the ordinary Town life of to-day, in short ; and are therefore, unable to take much active outdoor exercise :—*Not* for the healthy, living and exerting themselves vigorously all day long in the free open air of heaven. These thrice-blest individuals can digest—for a time,—not only any dinner they like to eat, but the table it is served on as well.

APPENDICES.

APPENDIX I.

WHEN I foresee (from worry, etc.) the probability of less sound sleep than I am used to under the Salisbury Treatment, I employ this means, which I hope others will find as effective as I do ; —premising, however, that I always rigidly abstain from fermentable foods at night.

On turning into bed, lie on the side on which you usually sleep, and get into a *perfectly restful and comfortable position.* Close not only your eyelids, but your eyes also, letting them follow the downward direction of the lids, and fixing your attention on keeping them down. Then, when the breathing has become quite gentle and regular, count softly to yourself, with no motion of the lips or sound at all, your respirations up to fifty.

Invariably long before I arrive at half that number I am lost in the enchanted fields of sleep,

and earth's joys, and cares, and sorrows, exist not·
for me.

If this fails, try wrapping a nice cold (not *too*)
wet towel round your head, with a dry one, folded,
over it. Bring it all well down over the brows
and the nape of the neck. An old-man's cotton
night-cap, shaped like an extinguisher, wrung out
of cold water, with a similar woollen dry one
over, makes a very satisfactory apparatus. This
is extremely soothing to the brain.

APPENDIX II.

I beg to say a few extra words to delicate people who are subject to catching chills or colds in throat and chest. To begin with, *you should always breathe through your nostrils, with shut lips ; never, sleeping or waking, through your mouth.* Taking this precaution will obviate breathing your own breath over again, further vitiated by the fluff from unnecessary woollen wraps over mouth and nose. And when you are out of doors, in spite of cold air,—nay, rather as protection *because* it is cold, with shoulders well thrown back, freely inhale the fresh, cold air through the nostrils, down to the very bottom of the chest. Inflate the lungs perfectly with it, then expel it slowly and thoroughly, and repeat the manœuvre again and again. Do it so constantly, when either walking or driving, that you will acquire *the habit of taking* these valuable lung-baths (always with closed mouth), so as to clear every hole and corner of the lungs, to fill *and sweep them out,* as *it were,* with pure, fresh air. You will thus widen and expand your chest, make yourself hardy

who have been delicate, and strong to withstand
even a severe climate and sudden alternations in
weather as the Salisbury patient should be.

If you are inadvertently caught in a damp,
cold atmosphere, without sufficient protection
against it, as may sometimes happen; your best
and surest chance of getting off scot-free, is
to continue these deep full breathings all the
while, with your mouth quite closed. I have
often saved myself severe after-suffering in similar situations, by this very simple expedient that
I am recommending to you : and while taking
·my lung-baths, I do not fear *now* being out in any
weather.

Shortly after beginning these large inspirations
regularly, your waistcoats and gown-bodies will
require letting out,—(*pace*, ladies, at the chest
only, *no tat the waist !*) to allow for the increase
of chest-girth. No weakly person need fear to
follow this advice and to banish muzzles —I
mean respirators, boas, clouds, and comforters in
cold weather, provided he or she always respires
through the nose and *not* through the mouth,
which was not intended by Nature as a breathing apparatus—which the nose clearly is. Please
remember this also that any sudden emotion, a

surprise of joy, or grief, or fear, excites the heart to beat dangerously fast, causing a horrid feeling of suffocation. Try and collect yourself in such a crisis sufficiently to take a succession of deep, full breaths; your courage and presence of mind will be rewarded by an immediate feeling of relief. I do not mention *anger* as a cause of violent emotion, for it would be too foolish to risk sudden death through a fit of passion, though one has heard of some so unhappy as to quit life in this unbecoming and precipitate fashion.

To return to chills and colds. If you have reason to believe that you have taken either seriously, and feel very wretched, shivery, and unable to get warm and comfortable again; *at once* take the following steps to nip it in the bud. Get some one to heat for you, a large blanket at the kitchen fire, bit by bit, rolling it up as it gets hot to retain the warmth. Strip entirely, lie down in bed, get wrapped quickly in this nice hot blanket from chin to feet, and have the bed-clothes (*minus the top* sheet) piled on. Have a piping hot bottle to your feet (with a flannel between you and the bottle), and other bottles at your sides, if you are not able to warm up quickly; and sip slowly (someone holding the cup for you) a large cupful of very hot, clear tea, or hot water. Presently you will be in a profuse perspiration, which, pray take the greatest care shall not get checked, and you will probably fall into a nice sound sleep, from which you may hope to wake up next morning all right, and ready for a good breakfast.

The same principle of Treatment, namely, to restore heat uniformly to the body, is to be pursued if you have taken something that has seriously disagreed with you, and causes you violent indigestion, such as, under some circumstances, ices, iced champagne, and iced milk may do,—or new bread, or pork, or any similar indigestible horror, only, in this latter case (of indigestion), besides the other hot bottles, one must be laid over the stomach, to help it by heat, to perform its needful task. Were it, however,—to let my fancy soar to poetic heights where I shall certainly never follow it,—my own case in which new bread, pork, iced anything played me this ill-natured turn,—I should not let the enemy torment me for hours, but should quickly rid myself of it by aid of a teaspoonful of antimonial wine; and then lie down, keep warm and quiet, sip the hot clear tea as a tonic, and make good resolutions for the future. Both these contingencies,—

the presence in the stomach of some stuff which
it is not able to digest, or a bad chill, are really
serious matters, and may have, if not sharply
taken in time, a decidedly awkward termination.
In regard to a chill, when you consider that the
outflow, perceptible or insensible, of the perspiration at the million pores all over the body, is
suddenly checked and thrown inward, it is easy
to understand the danger attending such a state
of things, nor is it surprising that it should cause
very serious illness, and even death. Try and induce a rapid and abundant flow again by every
means in your power, and those just detailed are,
I should say from experience, among the quickest
and safest. Be sure that in taking all reasonable
and judicious care of your health, you are showing yourself to be, not "molly-coddlish," but truly
wise and unselfish.

APPENDIX III.

The following case of one of my "Patients."
(whom I have never seen) is so instructive that I
am constrained to print a recent letter of his,
and I beg to call to your notice its great value
on several grounds, especially as so clearly showing, by his sudden decrease in weight, *that undigested food is worse than wasted*, and also that *the
manner of preparing the mince is of vital importance
to the complete success of the Treatment.*

About the middle of August last he was utterly broken down in health, and "had tried
many doctors in vain." He was feeble in body
and mind from his long ill-health, and had so
little vitality left, that he was unable to get warm
in bed, even with the help of hot bottles and
many blankets. Sleep had forsaken him, appetite had failed him, he could only partially digest
his food after great pain, and was greatly tor-
mented with flatulence and distention. For none
of these ills could he obtain relief.

He had been in this plight for nearly three years when he appealed to me for help. I at once advised him to go *strictly* on the Salisbury Treatment, which, with its reasons, I fully explained to him.

This he said he did, with fair results; yet not *so* good as I had expected. Therefore I *knew* he was tampering with it, and told him so. He replied that his friends were constantly dissuading him from the Treatment, and he himself was always wondering whether he had done really wisely in adopting it; so that while keeping to the diet and hot water which he felt were doing him good, he was, in addition, on his friends' advice, doing such and such things, and among them was wearing some kind of magnetic compress, which had brought out an eruption all round his body, and had greatly increased his weakness and general upset. In reply, I solemnly warned him that his health was in far too serious a state to bear tricks being played with it, and what was more, *I* would not bear them; that my responsibility was already grave enough in conducting him through the Salisbury Treatment at such a distance, and *this* responsibility I was willing to take. But that I emphatically refused to add to it the consequences of any experiments his friends might persuade him to try at the same time; and that he must either stick to the Treatment *alone* — or I must "withdraw from the case." (I often could not sleep at night from the anxiety this complicated responsibility caused me.) He promised strict fidelity to the Treatment in future, and much correspondence ensued. On December 27, 1888, he was able to report, " I am glad to inform you I am doing very well. I have dispensed now with hot bottles in bed at night, I sleep very much better, and friends are saying I am *looking* much better. . . . I have enjoyed myself to my heart's content this Xmas, a thing I would not have attempted last year or the year before. . . . I can say that the hot water and minced beef have done for me what all other so-called remedies failed to do. . . . I am so overjoyed to see myself going up in weight and feelings. . . ."

And now I come to his letter regarding the cooking of the mince and loss and regain of weight :—It is dated "April 6, 1889. In your letter of Thursday week you said as the reason why I was troubled with heartburn and flatulence again:—'Probably your mince is overcooked, and the great stumbling block thro' all the Treatment *is*, to get the mince just right.' This caused me to very particularly notice the state of the mince, with gratifying results. For some six weeks I have had my mince cooked in a *Bain Marie*, and ever since I have been troubled with heartburn and flatulence, and have gone down in weight 9 lbs. *Now* I have commenced upon the old plan, cooking in an ordinary saucepan, stirring constantly until the mince is *thoroughly hot* all through, and has lost its red color, remaining as soft as well-boiled rice—not hard and curly [that is a good word of his to describe the granular, gritty, conglobated lumps into which the mince forms when *too quickly* or *over* cooked] as it has been for six weeks. I digest this wonderfully, no trouble in any way whatever, heartburn and flatulence gone, weight risen in seven days 3¼ lbs., sleep improved, and I wake refreshed and ready for the day's work." And then he makes a very astute observation, to which I beg to call your particular attention, for it is entirely *true*. My intelligent patient continues : "The remedy of hot water and minced beef can be *defeated* by the mince being OVER COOKED. I have had a sim-

12

ilar experience with the *beef cakes*. Your plan of
the ordinary pan, stirring all the time, is the best,
I take daily note of my food, and it is by so doing that I can trace the evil and the hour it
commenced. I have got Mackenzie's digestive
wheaten biscuits, as you recommended, and they
are what you call delicious, in fact I could eat a
box of them a day, [!] they agree with me very
well ; so much so that I have had as many as six
at a time. [This addition to the beef diet has
been made only since he got well.] Some of
my friends who are in fair health have partially
gone on the Treatment with the object of preserving their health, seeing the wonderful change
it has made in me thro' your guidance and per-
sistency in urging me to keep on with the Treatment, and your earnest and repeated assurances
that all was well with me, in spite of very dark
days when I was inclined to give up and despair.
I could only see through a glass darkly then, full
of doubt and fears ; but now I can see the whole
thing clearly, and if I had to commence again, I
am sure I could get well in half the time it has
taken to get where I am now. I did things I
ought not to have done at times, and then friends
turned round and said it was the hot water."

So much for my satisfactory patient. When others write to me, "I cannot take to the mince," "I hate it," or "I am unable to digest the mince," I *know* that the lion in the path is simply that the mince is *too quickly* or *over* cooked, and I tell them so. In a short while, when all directions have been followed, I am told that it is eaten heartily, is "very nice," and that it gives no trouble either in eating or digesting. Once more please then, I repeat—the mince must be evenly mixed with cold water or stock, put in a saucepan, if over a hottish fire from ten to twelve minutes is sufficient to cook it, *stirring briskly all the while*—if over a colder fire it takes longer—but it is always *done, and must come off the fire the moment* that it is *thoroughly hot through*, and the *red* color has *changed to gray*. Its consistency before going on—and after coming off the fire, should be of a soft purée, more or less substantial or liquid, according as desired. Any deviation from this, renders the mince as insipid, indigestible, unassimilable and unpleasant, as good advice from a *true friend!*

April 9, 1889.   E. STUART.

APPENDIX IV.

· I CONFESS to being very sceptical myself in respect to a testimonial unverified by the writer's name and address, and do not, therefore, ask anyone to believe in the following extracts, albeit they are entirely genuine.

The reason they are anonymous is, that it was almost at the last moment the happy suggestion was made to me, that I should include them in my book "pour encourager les autres," and there was no time then to ask permission of the widely-scattered writers, who will, I fear, open their eyes a little, at thus suddenly encountering their own words.

Will my kind correspondents—known and unknown—graciously pardon the freedom I have used, and indulgently accept my hearty thanks for this their good help in furthering the cause? As some amends for withholding from publicity the names and addresses of my correspondents, I have been careful to furnish *the dates.*

INDIVIDUAL TESTIMONY CONCERNING THE SALISBURY
TREATMENT.

A busy City friend writes : " February, 1888.
I have stuck religiously to my two pints a day,
and have wonderfully benefited thereby ; have
conquered the heartburn, indigestion, and the
constant headaches I used to suffer from. I have
minced beef, cooked according to your instructions, three times a week at least, and find it a
great comfort on my arrival at home, tired out
with hard work. I am *much* better, many grateful thanks to you."

A lady from abroad writes : " February, 1888.
What with the bad food and constant chills, I
should have had a regular illness this winter but
for the hot water. . . . —— and his family
all take it now, and I hand on to you the blessings they send me." [I wish " blessings " were
substantial things ! E. S.]

Another City friend writes : " April, 1888. Regarding the minced collops, I do feel so grateful
to you for your suggestion. When I come home
jaded and tired out, brain and body, and feeling
as if I could not *touch* food, I can always eat with

much enjoyment, a nice dish of the mince, and feel so well, and light, and *rested*, all the evening afterward. The hot water too, has done me a very great amount of good in many ways.".

A gentleman at the Antipodes writes: "January, 1889. I haven't had *one* bad night since I began my hot water. . . . and I am much encouraged by other good signs to go on with it."

A gentleman who *was* thoroughly out of health writes: "December, 1888. I am still on the Treatment, and am *much* benefited thereby. . . I will cheerfully continue the Treatment, being greatly encouraged by my improvement." The same gentleman reports: "March, 1889. I am wonderfully better in every way when I keep to the rules of living" [he is not on the *strict* diet].

A lady writes: "October, 1888. Nor must I forget to mention the servant who saw your pamphlet on the drawing-room table, read it, and picked herself up from really bad health, entirely by following it."

A lady writes: "October, 1888. I am feeling *ever* so much better for the hot water, and have

quite a fine complexion now. Cook, who has suffered from eczema for years, and has been to nu-
merous doctors without deriving any benefit, has
taken to the hot water, and says she is feeling already immensely better for it."

A lady, after narrating the benefit various suf-
ferers had derived from following the advice in
my small pamphlet, adds : "As for —— I haven't
seen her with so good and clear a complexion as
now, since she was a girl—all hot water."

A lady writes (no date), 1888: "My sister is
keeping wonderfully well, thanks to you and hot
water. I have not seen her eat so heartily and
with such enjoyment for many years, and she
looks so well too."

An invalid old lady writes (no date, but it was
in autumn), 1888 : "The treatment has done me
a *power* of good. The very first day I felt a decided improvement, and my night was excellent."
And a few months later, this same lady writes :
"I may say I improve *daily* but gradually, and
now I do look forward to getting about again before long, thanks to your advice. I am able to
keep pretty rigidly to my diet too."

An old lady writes : "January, 1889. I have derived *very great* benefit from the Salisbury Treatment."

A gentleman from the far side of our Planet, writes, toward the end of 1888 : "On receipt of your pamphlet, I began the hot water with enthusiasm. *At once* there was an improvement . . . and already I have derived much benefit from the hot water in other ways too ; and feel sure it will do everybody good."

A lady writes : "January, 1889. I cannot express how grateful I am to hot water and all it has done for me. Mrs. C. gave me one of your pamphlets not quite a year ago, and I have stuck to the hot water-drinking night and morning ever since, and feel *years* younger in consequence, and those whom I have persuaded to take it regularly, tell me how much it has done for them too."

A gentleman who was in a very broken-down condition and very sorry for himself writes : "April, 1888. I have tried the exclusive diet of minced beef, and hot water four times a day for a month now, with the best results. Quite free

from the miseries undergone from indigestion, I
may say, for years past. Though weak for the
first few days, yet experienced a new sensation
of lightness from the time I began the Treatment,
and an absence of the sense of oppression and
frequent pain after meals. Sleep, sounder and
more refreshing. Increased facility in walking
and mounting hills. Freedom from palpitation
and pain in the region of the heart. Marked effect
of hot water in relieving exhaustion, preventing
any wish for liquids at meals, and quenching all
desire for stimulants ; besides creating a hearty
appetite, especially for breakfast. Exclusive meat
diet unquestionably most easily and rapidly digested, causing no subsequent discomfort. So far
from palling on me, the taste for it has rather
grown. . . . "

A lady, who knows my own former pitiable
condition, writes : "March, 1889. *You* are a
splendid advertisement for the Salisbury Treatment. . . . The very simplicity of it makes
people incredulous ; but I also can speak from
experience of the good it does. I have taken the
hot water steadily for about three years, and have
not had, during that time, a single liver attack,

and in many ways, am in much better health. Indeed I am very well and strong now, and feel I
owe you a deal of gratitude for having persuaded me to try the hot water."

A gentleman writes : "April, 1889. One good
the hot water has done me is, that I simply *love*
my meals." [Considering that the writer is one of
the most popular diners-out, and that his meals at
the time of writing, consisted mainly of minced
beef, this seems pretty telling in favor of the virtues of hot water.] "I have no particular feeling
of hunger, but when I sit down, I just delight in
my food. Another good it has done me, is, that
I have quite lost an inclination to be stout under
my waistcoat, a great improvement, if I were
younger and could care for that."

A lady writes : "March, 1889. The hot water is
doing my little boy good."

A gentleman who had been very ill indeed, and
whom I had helped by letter, writes : "March,
1889. I got your book on Monday week, and
have read it through several times with profit, in
fact I cannot let it out of my hands it is so inter-

eating. . . . The best judges of your book
and the System, are those who *suffer*, or who
have suffered, and have put same to a test, among
whom I class myself. . . . My friends say
I am looking very much better, fuller in the
face, and they can bear witness how at first, it
seemed to pull me down ; now they see that
the Salisbury Treatment is a *building up* of the
frame. . . . I am a different man from
what I was a short time ago, prior to commencing the hot water and mínced beef. . . . I
will post you up in my state and progress. If I
go back now, it will be my own fault."

A lady writes : "April, 1889. . . . The doctors put me on a very generous diet [!] eggs,
milk, cream, farinaceous puddings, etc., etc. In
consequence, the rheumatism has returned, indigestion, biliousness, acidity. . . . have been
making my life miserable ;—when I fortunate-
ly came across your book. I have been following the advice about diet and drinking the hot
water four times a day, but I cannot take more
than ⅓ a pint as a rule, sometimes ¼, but the pint
seems too much for me. . . . I have tak-
en the minced beef three times a day with *a little*

crisp toast, for a fortnight. . . . I am decidedly better, and have *nearly* lost the rheumatism, but still feel indigestion and biliousness
slightly. . . ." I replied, counselling perseverance. This lady writes again: "April 11,
1889. I take *the pint* of hot water night and morning now, but have not been able to do so in the
middle of the day yet. I have been feeling much
better since I wrote, the rheumatism is now nothing to speak of, the dull aching pain in my chest
and pit of stomach with heat, is much relieved.
I still have at times aching in the middle of the
back between the shoulder blades, which seems
very much like flatulence. . . ." Same lady:
"April 24, 1889. Thank you very much for sending me the paper about your patient, it is very very
cheering. You will be glad to hear" [I was more
than glad, E. S.] "that I am *much* better than
when I last wrote to you. I followed your advice,
and 'thought it out for myself'—and found the
mince had not been cooked properly—too long
done, and not stirred all the time. I can assure
you I *hated* it. Now it is only cooked about ten
minutes and stirred *briskly*. It is very nice and
I enjoy it. . . . I have kept strictly to the
mince and a few of Mackenzie's wheaten biscuits,

although my friends keep telling me I *look* paler and thinner, and want me to take a more mixed diet. But I do not heed them. I can now take my four pints of hot water a day " [Bravo ! E. S.] "My rheumatism is *gone ;* and the indigestion and flatulence are much better. I feel stronger altogether. . . . I cannot feel grateful enough to you and your book for helping me so much . . . Many of my friends have got the book, and take the hot water and *partial* diet, and express themselves so pleased at feeling so much better."

A gentleman with whom I have been in correspondence on his health, for some months, writes from very far away : "April, 1889. . . . I have just been dining with our new governor, Sir —— and Lady ——, and was very fully on the 'Spree,' but you allow that sometimes." [It's a poor heart that *never* rejoices ! E. S.] "I am glad, however, to report that what with champagne and other comestibles taken at dinner, no hurt to digestion followed, and I attribute this to the now healthy state of the organs. I am constantly preaching the minced beef and hot water."

A lady writes : " May, 1889. I used to suffer a good deal from biliousness and sick headaches, but since by your advice, beginning the hot water, I am thankful to say I have got rid of both. Though quite well now, I still continue the morning and evening pints, and would be very sorry to leave them off."

A gentleman writes : " May, 1889. If ever I am conscious that I am selfish, it is when asked by a friend to lend your book ! I know you will be pleased to hear I have converted many, with whom I come in contact daily. Not the least interesting case is that of Mr. ——, who was frequently detained at home on account of illness. I lent him your book, he felt he was bad enough to commence the System ; and since, he says, he has felt *very well*, and thanks me for making it known to him. He is so in earnest about it, that he has a small kettle at his office, which he heats on a gas stand, and enjoys his potation in the midst of his official work. I too have adopted this plan in my office. I have also bought a mincer, for I do enjoy a good dish of mince for my evening meal, after a stiff day of mental and physical work. Being fond of athletics, I bicycle a good deal, and find the sustaining power of the well-digested minced beef, beyond that of any other form of nourishment I have ever tried. Also, in hot weather, for thirst in cycling, I have found that the hot water with a squeeze of lemon is most effective in *stopping* the thirst, and *refreshing* one thoroughly."

The following testimony from a gentleman is valuable, not only as a record of his own improvement, but, to thoughtful minds, for the broadside-light it throws on the suitability of *minced* food in semi-starvation—(which means *weakness*—and which would equally apply to a case of exhaustion from any cause whatever), and also, as showing how this Treatment does away with the need of, or desire for, stimulant. "May, 1889. . . . First let me *assure* you that I am very *much* better. It is observed by everyone, and many friends have already begun the hot water, and some the diet. One very stout man has already lessened his obesity, and, what is more, has got rid of an affection in the knee which his doctor could not cure, and he now walks well. . . . Your book should have a

great sale and do a world of good. A matron of
a great London hospital told me yesterday, that
she had to prepare *mince* for 50 children every
day, who are put upon that diet after half starvation. I am sure this system will be a great Tem-
perance agent, besides other good things, for it
seems to do away with all craving for alcoholics.
I shall try and get some to reform their drinking habits with it. I never touch wine now, nor
want it, my one glass which I took is really unnecessary, and I have stopped it. . . . The
food when I wake in the night is delightful, and
sends me to sleep at once." (This is what I call
a most satisfactory and first-rate Patient, taking
an intelligent interest in the Treatment, and
looking at it outside of his own case. E. S.)

A lady writes: "May, 1889. . . . I am
much indebted to your book and have derived
one great benefit from drinking the hot water. I
have had rheumatic gout all my life more or less,
. . . the ache I used to suffer from continually
has left me, and I find much less difficulty in getting my boots on. . . . I take a good supper
of mince at 8. I have only tried your system for
about six weeks. Your book will help many to

better health, if they will only persevere in following it."

A lady writes : "July, 1889. I feel I must let you know the benefit I am deriving from the hot water and beef diet as set forth in your book on Dr. Salisbury's Treatment. I have been ill for nearly two years, suffering from dyspepsia, nervous exhaustion. . . . The suffering has been terrible, and my recovery seemed so protracted that I had begun to despair of ever feeling well again. . . . I have now lived on the minced beef and a *little* toast and butter for a month, and am feeling quite different . . . and there are many other encouraging signs of improvement in my health. I went to some German Baths last August, but did not derive as much benefit from them, as I have from this beef diet and hot water after little more than a month's trial."

I close the list with a pleasant word from a very dear French friend : "November, 1888. Je prends ma petite tasse d'eau chaude, tous les jours à 4 heures, en souvenir de vous ; j'ai même invité Mme C. à venir vendredi, se joindre à nous, dans ce repas aquatique !"

13

I regret that I cannot give my best and most telling Testimonials, having always sent them straight off to Dr. Salisbury to rejoice *his* heart too. These however which I have quoted out of an *immense number*, are quite sufficient to prove that, once started on the right road of the Salisbury Treatment, you, who went forth with weeping, shall come again with gladness, bringing your sheaves with you.

> " Joyous as when the reapers bear
> The harvest treasure home ! "

APPENDIX V.

In July, 1889, I met with a very serious tricycle
accident, because, feeling quite ridiculously and
buoyantly well, my riding became rash and fool-
hardy. I smashed my ribs on the left side and
was a good deal knocked about in other directions. A doctor at once examined me, and another five days later, for I was sure that at least
one rib was broken, from the great pain, and the
impossibility of breathing except in short gasps,
also from a slight grating I heard and felt on
moving. Both doctors asserted after investigation that I was quite sound and only very badly
bruised internally. They urged remedies upon
me, and "something to soothe the pain," all which
I rejected, though assured that I should have fever
and inflammation, and general disturbance of the
system from the accident. This I did not for a
moment believe to be compatible with the very
healthy way in which I had for so long fed.

I at once returned to the strict Salisbury diet,

and increased my four pints a day to six. The
result more than justified my confidence. For
I had not one degree's rise in temperature, no fever nor inflammation, nor the least derangement
in any one way whatever : while my nights from
the first, in spite of exceeding pain and impeded breathing, were uniformly lovely, with many
hours of sound refreshing sleep. I *felt so well in
health* too, the whole time I was laid up.

Nearly a fortnight after the accident (during
which time I had to make a short railway journey, rising from bed to do it), on the pain becoming altogether unbearable, I sent for an eminent
bone-setter ; who found one rib broken and another badly splintered. These he set to rights,
to the music of my vociferous yells. He was
amazed to find me in first-rate health, after so
much pain, and the fortnight's neglect of the injury,—and could not understand the absence of inflammation, and there being no systemic derangement in any way. I explained the reason, and
the Salisbury Treatment, with the value of which
he was greatly impressed, and he began at once
to test the virtues of hot water on himself for
liver, reporting in a few days his great improvement and relief.

Now the sole reason why I have related this untoward experience is this. On the third day, I was, unfortunately, at my early dinner, tempted to take a tablespoonful of rice and milk pudding (made without sugar) which, if I had been going about as usual, would not, for a time or two have hurt me. In about half an hour the pains in my back and side became all at once terribly acute, and my breathing much more hampered. Dr. Salisbury has taught me to look for the cause of any relapse, in something *I myself* have done or left undone; so I searched assiduously now, and thought carefully over the last few hours. Ere long it flashed upon me that the rice pudding was the culprit, and that the sudden oncome of very acute pain, was simply due to *flatulence; from the wind or gas* generated by the ferment-able farinaceous pudding, *pressing upon the injured parts inside.*

Into half a pint of warm water, I stirred a large teaspoonful of bicarbonate of soda, and drank it in big sips. This had the desired effect of immediately raising a great quantity of sour flatus, and at each eructation the relief to the internal pains, was great, while my breathing became perceptibly easier. When I had finished the hot water and soda, I took, sipping slowly, one and one-half to two pints of plain hot water (it was then about 7.30 P.M.). Sour flatus continued to rise for about two hours more, each time giving relief to the pain ; and my night's sleep was undisturbed. I studiously eschewed fermentable food till I was well again, and daily made good and rapid progress, on my exclusive diet of minced beef, *at the same time causing six pints a day of pure, fresh warm water to traverse the bruised and wounded tissues.*

Now the moral of the whole matter is this. Farinaceous and milk puddings, and similar foods, are erroneously recommended for nearly all weakly persons, more or less ill, as "light, wholesome, and nourishing." I long ago, by actual and repeated trial, proved to my entire conviction, that their lightness and nourishing properties are a snare and delusion ; and I have just now given my experience of—*under certain circumstances*—their " wholesomeness."

I do NOT, *for one moment*, intend to say that farinaceous puddings, etc., are harmful to all people, and at all times,—to the healthy, or even to the only fairly healthy, taken in moderation ; but I do emphatically say this,—as the lesson learned from many carefully observed experiments, and I maintain it,—that for those with weak digestions and in delicate health, all such foods *are distinctly hurtful,* their "lightness and nourishing properties" are *not* a small third those of beef and mutton ; whilst the gas engendered by fermentation, is safe to cause *some* upset to the delicate invalid (although not, probably, like mine, aggravated by internal injuries), and this upset, slight or grave, will be laid at any door but the right one. Then, things are given to ease the sudden pain, and allay malaise (which are credited to the illness), but sedatives and anodynes, *while the unsuspected cause is continued,* can do no lasting good : and the mischief done by *them* to the invalid, can scarcely be overrated. I repeat :—All I have said has no reference to robust people, who may be left to take care of themselves,—I am speaking, earnestly speaking, in the interests solely of *invalids, great or partial,* whether bedridden or not.

INDEX.

Heartily, always eat, 38.
Hogs, experiments on, 19, 20, 163.
Hogs cannot safely "make hogs of themselves," 163.
Hot water, alone is beneficial, 149.
Hot water benefits everybody, 27, 149.
Hot water cures dipsomania, 93.
Hot water comforts and relieves, 138.
Hot water cures indigestion, etc., 25.
Hot water helps to soothe worry, 102, 103.
Hot water increases vitality and circulation, 26.
Hot water inimical to suicide, 91.
Hot water is an internal bath, 25, 27.
Hot water makes for health, 28.
Hot water, nausea fancied from, 24.
Hot water, objects and uses of, 25, 27.
Hot water produces sleep, 27.
Hot water, quantity to be taken, 22.
Hot water quenches thirst, best of all drinks, 24.
Hot water removes tendency to catch colds and chills, 26.
Hot water, right times for taking, 22.
Hot water strengthens and soothes nerves, 27.
Hot water, temperature of, 22.
Hot water, temperature in hemorrhage, 138.
Hot water, to be taken in all illnesses, 150.
Hot water, to be taken *along with* the diet, 150.

Hours, five between meals, 65.
Hours, for food, 22.
Hours, for hot water, 22.
How to keep well, 90.
Hungry in the night, 39.
Hurry never; "go slowly," 56.

I.

Ice a medicine, not a food, 138.
Ill-health, we bring on ourselves, 127.
Illnesses, cure for, 152.
Illnesses, preventable, 61.
Illnesses, produced by unhealthy alimentation, 95, 133, 163.
Illnesses, severe, treatment cures, 152.
Illnesses, slight, treatment cures, 148, 149.
Incurable diseases shown to be curable, 121, 122, 123, 125, 130.
Indigestion, cure of, 25.
Indigestion, effects of, 155.
Infections a permissible cause of illness, 121.
Inflammatory diseases, 128.
Injuries likewise are so, 121.
Insoluble bodies not to be swallowed, 71.
Instructions to be exactly followed, 57.
Intelligence imperatively demanded, 38, 55.
Intelligent observation, advantage of, 55, 74.

L.

Last meal chiefly a meat one, 82, 155.
Last meal entirely a meat one, 155.
Lemon-juice, substitute for vinegar, 24, 34.

A HOUSEHOLD REMEDY.

In every family there should be some remedy for the speedy removing of inflammation, as this is the immediate cause of nine-tenths of the aches, pains, and annoyances to which the physical body is subject. By treating these different troubles at their commencement with some efficacious medicament, you get rid of the cause, and it is then an easy matter for nature to restore the diseased parts to a normal condition. If the proper remedy is on hand, to be used in cases of emergency, days of misery are often averted.

COMPOUND MENTHOL ICE

is positively the grandest, the most wonderful, and truly marvelous

HOUSEHOLD REMEDY

ever prescribed by a physician and dispensed by a pharmacist.

It has been used on prescriptions for a number of years, and its great power for combat-

1

ing·the evils produced by that common enemy —inflammation—became so well known, its value so firmly established and so well sustained, that in the short time it has been before the public its merits have carried it to the front. The following sentence heads the circular describing this remedy: "We challenge the world for an ointment, salve, or liniment that will do *as much*, and do it *as well*." This claim is far-reaching, but it is justified by the actual results obtained from its use, as thousands have attested. Without doubt CATARRH is one of the most common and most annoying ailments of the present time, probably five-sixths of the people in this country being afflicted with it in some form. This need not and would not be, if every one used Compound Menthol Ice faithfully, it being almost a specific for this malady. The beneficial effects are realized on the first application, as the air passages are opened, the head cleared, and it is easily kept in that condition.

Such expressions as this are very often heard after using the Ice the first time: "I have not breathed through my nose before for days, but now it is perfectly free, and my head feels good."

HAY FEVER and **ROSE COLD** are possibly more annoying troubles while they last than **CATARRH**, but half of the cases can be prevented entirely, and the other half can be modified so that life is not a burden. As a preventive, the Ice should be used fully a month previous to the expected attack.

PILES, in any of its forms, is a most distressing complaint, but a remedy can now be had which will effect a cure in nearly every case, and for this trouble as well as all others, one does not have to wait weeks for results: relief is experienced at once.

ERYSIPELAS, ECZEMA, SALT RHEUM, HIVES, and **SKIN DISEASES** of all kinds are rapidly and permanently cured by using the Ice. The itching or burning sensation attending diseases of this class is immediately allayed, and the skin soon assumes its natural condition.

SORES, and especially those of a *chronic* nature, are quickly healed by wrapping the parts in the Ice. **PIMPLES** on the **FACE,**

3

CHAPPED HANDS and LIPS, CUTS, BURNS, TENDER and FROST-BITTEN FEET, should all be treated with Compound Menthol Ice, as it is without a rival for combating all the troubles induced by inflammation.

This remedy is especially valuable for children's use, and particularly so for breaking up those COLDS or SNUFFLES, which is the starting point for a chronic case of CATARRH. Mothers, use the right remedy at the right time, and save your children endless days of suffering.

This preparation is a veritable medicine-chest, and no mistake is made in the claim that it is

A HOUSEHOLD REMEDY.

There is constant inquiry for some simple remedy that will "break up" or cure a COLD in the HEAD—something that will act at once and prove efficient in every case. Those who read this article need not make further inquiries, as

COMPOUND MENTHOL POWDER

is the right preparation to use, its merits being recognized by a multitude of people. It is a non-sneezing, non-irritating powder. It allays the inflammation, kills whatever germs there

4

may be—in fact, removes the *cause* of the trouble, nature does the rest. By using this Powder faithfully the most severe **COLD** in the **HEAD** can be "broken up" inside of twenty-four hours, and what is especially gratifying, its agreeable effect is realized immediately. Its virtue lies not alone in its ability to cure, it is a preventive as well.

HEADACHE is relieved by the first inhalation of this *Powder*. As a remedy for **CLEARING** the **HEAD** and **THROAT** it has no equal, and public speakers and singers are using it all over the country, and hearty words of praise are they bestowing upon it. Its wonderfully *refreshing* effect makes it a valuable agent to use in cases of **FAINTING**, it being far superior to "Smelling Salts" for crowded and ill-ventilated rooms. It is so convenient and so pleasant to use, and as such a remedy is in constant demand, it is only a question of time when its use will be universal.

Your attention is now called to another preparation which is equally as beneficial for *its* purpose as Compound Menthol Ice and Compound Menthol Powder are for their's.

5

This one is

COMPOUND MENTHOL DROPS,

and is used for all troubles of the THROAT and BRONCHIAL TUBES. A HACKING COUGH yields to its action without a struggle. THAT TICKLING in the THROAT is quickly subdued by its influence. A SORE THROAT is brought to subjection in a very short time, even when there are plenty of cankers to be seen. What is true of one remedy is equally true of the three: they contain no opiate of any nature, are perfectly harmless, and very agreeable to use.

Rev. A. H. Clapp, D.D., Treasurer American Home Missionary Society, No. 34 Bible House, New York City, says:

"You may use my name in any way you choose to further the sale of your very valuable Compound Menthol Remedies. I have used the preparations to my entire satisfaction (Drops in particular) and can heartily recommend them as being worthy the confidence of the public."

These Remedies are being mailed to all parts of the country by the proprietors, KELLOGG & HITCHCOCK Co., 4 Park Place, New York City, the Ice on receipt of 50c.; the Powder and Drops on receipt of 25c. each.

6

1730 BROADWAY, NEW YORK.

Having called the attention of the profession to Menthol and its preparations in several Medical Journals, and having at the request of a Japanese official made a report on the uses of Menthol to the Japanese Government, through His Excellency the Hon. R. Kuki, Minister resident at Washington, I felt that my knowledge of the value of Menthol warranted me in suggesting to you the desirability of making it a household remedy, and I think it is not derogatory in me to enforce my recommendation of your preparations of this article. Certainly I should not now endorse your "Compounds," had I not confidence in your character and in the Menthol. Yours truly,

Ephraim Cutter, m. d.

BROOKLYN.

I found your "Compound Menthol Powder" gave me immediate relief, both from a severe headache and a cold in my head. I cheerfully testify to its efficacy and value. Yours faithfully,

Fredrick Warde

OPERA HOUSE, CLEVELAND, O.

Your "Compound Menthol Powder" has proved very efficacious.

7

I have the pleasure of inf...
sonally tried the "Compoun...
it beneficial, as well as ver...
not prevented my annual a...
held it in check to a certain...
comfort. Please send me a...
tion.

The "Compound Mentho...
excellent results, and can r...
with a severe cold. Believe...

Jen...

HARRIGAN'S PARK TH...
BROADWAY AND 35TH...
Edward Harrigan, Prop'r.   M. W.

I found your "Compound...
for a cold in the head, and...
tion, I would cheerfully re...
professionals.   Respect...

Edw...

8

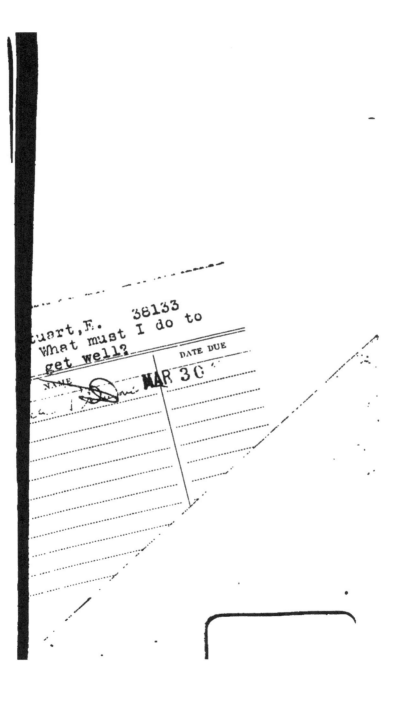

tuart,F.   38133
What must I do to
get well?

NAME   DATE DUE

MAR 30

I have the pleasure of informing you that I have personally tried the "Compound Menthol Ice," and found it beneficial, as well as very agreeable to use. It has not prevented my annual attack of hay fever, but has held it in check to a certain degree, and promoted my comfort. Please send me another bottle of the preparation.

C. C. Dawson,

Sec'y U. S. Hay Fever Ass'n.

NEW YORK.

The "Compound Menthol Powder" I have used with excellent results, and can recommend it to all suffering with a severe cold. Believe me, respectfully yours,

Jannauschek

HARRIGAN'S PARK THEATRE,
BROADWAY AND 35TH ST.
Edward Harrigan, Prop'r.   M. W. Hanley, Manager.

NEW YORK.

I found your "Compound Menthol Powder" excellent for a cold in the head, and as actors dread that affliction, I would cheerfully recommend it to my brother professionals.   Respectfully,

Edward Harrigan

DISTRICT ATTORNEY'S OFFICE, COUNTY OF CORTLAND,
CORTLAND, N. Y.

This is to certify that I have used your "Compound Menthol Ice" in my family for catarrh and head colds, with the most satisfactory results. I can cheerfully recommend it to the public.

H. L. Brown

District Attorney.

——————

BROOKLYN, N. Y.

Your "Compound Menthol Powder" found me with a cold, and I immediately tested its efficacy with favorable results. It will, I am sure, prove a blessing to players, preachers, and all other public entertainers, who may have the good fortune to use it.

Stuart Robson

——————

HOWE & HUMMEL,
COUNSELLORS-AT-LAW.

NEW YORK.

I have used your "Compound Menthol Powder" with great benefit. It has on several occasions relieved me from severe hoarseness, and it is a valuable aid to public speakers. From the great benefit I have derived from it, I have recommended it to several of my legal friends who speak most highly of it. I shall never be without it.

Yours respectfully,

William F. Howe

9

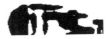

THE GAGE CUTTER WOOD M'F'G CO.,
HOMER, N. Y.

I have personally used your "Compound Menthol Ice" for catarrh, and beneficial results were so quickly obtained, and have been so permanent, that I would advise every sufferer with this obnoxious disease to immediately procure a jar of the "Ice," and use it faithfully. In our family we consider the "Ice" an indispensable household remedy.

A. S. Gage.

BURROUGH BROS. M'F'G CO.,
BALTIMORE, MD.

I have used your "Compound Menthol Ice" for rose cold and hay fever during this entire season, and with my own experience before me, sincerely believe that the faithful application of this valuable remedy will afford complete relief from these most miserable of diseases.

Horace Burrough

NEW YORK.

I have found your "Compound Menthol Powder" to be a useful and refreshing preparation for cold in the head and for irritation of the throat.

Yours respectfully,

Abram S. Hewitt

10

WILMINGTON, DEL.

I have personally received great benefit from your "Compound Menthol Powder," and warmly recommend its use in cases of cold in the head, neuralgia, etc.

Yours very truly,

Maggie Mitchell

NEW YORK.

I received your bottle of "Compound Menthol Powder" at a moment when I was suffering from an aggravated nasal and bronchial irritation, contracted by coming out of a superheated audience-room and standing in an east wind to converse with a friend. I had tried all the chlorates and all the astringents without relief. Your powder acted instantly, and I am bound to tell you has cured me. I never found anything so grateful to an excoriated membrane as the Menthol Powder. You can use this in any way you choose.

A. C. Wheeler

(Nym Crinkle.)

MEMPHIS, TENN.

Your "Compound Menthol Powder" has afforded me great relief from hoarseness. Travelling, as I do, the change of climate ofttimes affects my throat, and your remedy certainly acts quick and effective.

Respectfully yours,

Kate Castleton

11

I frankly answer your letter of inquiry just received. I have been a great sufferer from Hay Fever for more than twenty-five years. It is never attended with asthma. It comes promptly about the 20th of August and continues until the appearance of frost. I have never found any relief in medicine worth speaking of until last summer. Sojourning at Bethlehem in the White Mountains for two or three months each year, I escaped the attack, but I have an impression that the exemption is only temporary, and I think that I have stronger catarrhal tendencies in the Fall and Winter.

I have a doubt whether it is wise to seek exemption by change of locality, especially when the Hay Fever is not attended by asthma.

Last year I did not go to the White Mountains, but spent two or three months in the northwestern corner of Rhode Island near the Massachusetts line. I had little or no Hay Fever, certainly not more than I have had on "HAY FEVER DAYS" in the White Mountains. Strange to say, I have less difficulty this winter with catarrh and colds in the head than for many years before.

The place of my sojourn in Rhode Island last summer I know is not one of the "exempted places," for on previous occasions I have suffered extremely in that locality.

I attribute my escape from Hay Fever attack last summer mainly to the free use of "Compound Menthol Ice," prepared by KELLOGG & HITCHCOCK CO., of New York. I regard this preparation as one of the most wonderful discoveries of the age. I cannot say too much for it as a remedy for all diseases of the "HAY FEVER" variety, and freely recommend it to my friends, and propose to give it another thorough trial next season.

R. B. WESTBROOK, D.D., LL.D.,
1707 Oxford Street.